T0226803

Ethics in Psychiatry

Editors

REBECCA WEINTRAUB BRENDEL
MICHELLE HUME

PSYCHIATRIC CLINICS OF NORTH AMERICA

www.psych.theclinics.com

Consulting Editor
HARSH K. TRIVEDI

December 2021 • Volume 44 • Number 4

ELSEVIER

1600 John F. Kennedy Boulevard • Suite 1800 • Philadelphia, Pennsylvania, 19103-2899

http://www.theclinics.com

PSYCHIATRIC CLINICS OF NORTH AMERICA Volume 44, Number 4
December 2021 ISSN 0193-953X, ISBN-13: 978-0-323-83568-8

Editor: Lauren Boyle
Developmental Editor: Diana Ang

Psychiatric Clinics of North America (ISSN 0193-953X) is published quarterly by Elsevier Inc., 360 Park Avenue South, New York, NY 10010-1710. Months of issue are March, June, September, and December. Business and Editorial Offices: 1600 John F. Kennedy Blvd., Suite 1800, Philadelphia, PA 19103-2899. Periodicals postage paid at New York, NY and additional mailing offices. Subscription prices are $338.00 per year (US individuals), $966.00 per year (US institutions), $100.00 per year (US students/residents), $406.00 per year (Canadian individuals), $499.00 per year (international individuals), $1024.00 per year (Canadian & international institutions), and $220.00 per year (international students/residents), $100.00 per year (Canadian & students/residents). Foreign air speed delivery is included in all *Clinics'* subscription prices. All prices are subject to change without notice. **POSTMASTER:** Send address changes to *Psychiatric Clinics of North America*, Elsevier Health Sciences Division, Subscription Customer Service, 3251 Riverport Lane, Maryland Heights, MO 63043. **Customer Service: 1-800-654-2452 (US). From outside the United States, call 1-314-447-8871. Fax: 1-314-447-8029. E-mail: journalscustomerservice-usa@elsevier.com (for print support) and journalsonlinesupport-usa@elsevier.com (for online support).**

Reprints. For copies of 100 or more, of articles in this publication, please contact the Commercial Reprints Department, Elsevier Inc., 360 Park Avenue South, New York, New York 10010-1710. Tel.: 212-633-3874, Fax: 212-633-3820, E-mail: reprints@elsevier.com.

Psychiatric Clinics of North America is covered in *MEDLINE/PubMed (Index Medicus), Current Contents/Social and Behavioral Sciences, Social Science Citation Index, Embase/Excerpta Medica,* and PsycINFO.

Contributors

CONSULTING EDITOR

HARSH K. TRIVEDI, MD, MBA
President and Chief Executive Officer, Sheppard Pratt Health System, Baltimore, Maryland

EDITORS

REBECCA WEINTRAUB BRENDEL, MD, JD
Associate Director, Center for Bioethics, Director, Master of Bioethics Degree Program, Assistant Professor of Psychiatry, Harvard Medical School, Director of Law and Ethics, Center for Law, Brain, and Behavior, Department of Psychiatry, Massachusetts General Hospital, Boston, Massachusetts

MICHELLE HUME, MD, PhD
Forensic Psychiatrist, Mendota Mental Health Institute, Madison, Wisconsin

AUTHORS

MELISSA ABRAHAM, PhD, MSc
Director, Psychologist, Faculty Associate, Associate Faculty, Research Ethics Consultation Unit, Division of Clinical Research, Department of Psychiatry, Massachusetts General Hospital, Center for Bioethics, Harvard Medical School, Ariadne Labs

SAFIAH AMARA, MD
Psychiatrist, Northeast Ohio Medical University, Rootstown, Ohio

LAURA BRIZ, MD
Psychiatrist, Eating Recovery Center/Pathlight, Chicago, Illinois

BETHANY BRUMBAUGH, BA
Student, Harvard Medical School, Boston, Massachusetts

AMANDA CALHOUN, MD, MPH
Child and Adolescent Fellow, Yale Child Study Center, New Haven, Connecticut

PHILIP J. CANDILIS, MD, DFAPA
Director of Medical Affairs, Co-Director of the Forensic Psychiatry Fellowship, Saint Elizabeths Hospital, Washington, DC, DC Department of Behavioral Health, Professor of Psychiatry, The George Washington University School of Medicine & Health Sciences, Washington, DC

SEAN D. CLEARY, PhD, MPH
Associate Professor, Department of Epidemiology, Milken Institute School of Public Health, The George Washington University, Washington, DC

RACHEL CONRAD, MD
Department of Psychiatry, Instructor of Psychiatry, Harvard Medical School, Faculty, Harvard Medical School Center for Bioethics, Child and Adolescent Psychiatrist, Brigham and Women's Hospital, Boston, Massachusetts

CHARLES C. DIKE, MD, MPH, FRCPsych
Associate Professor of Psychiatry, Yale University School of Medicine, New Haven, Connecticut

BRANDON HAMM, MD, MS
Department of Psychiatry and Behavioral Sciences, Northwestern University, Chicago, Illinois

MARTA D. HERSCHKOPF, MD, MSt
Instructor, Part-Time, Department of Psychiatry, Attending Psychiatrist, Beth Israel Deaconess Medical Center, Harvard Medical School, Faculty, Harvard Medical School Center for Bioethics, Boston, Massachusetts

KELSEY HOBART, MD
Psychiatry Resident, Saint Elizabeths Hospital, DC Department of Behavioral Health, Washington, DC

MICHELLE HUME, MD, PhD
Forensic Psychiatrist, Mendota Mental Health Institute, Madison, Wisconsin

VENKATA R. JONNALAGADDA, MD, DFAPA, DFAACAP
Associate Chief of Staff, Greenville VA Health Care Center, Durham VA Healthcare System, Departments of Psychiatric Medicine and Pediatrics, Assistant Professor, East Carolina University School of Medicine, Greenville, North Carolina

KRISTEN LOHSE, PsyD
Psychologist, ACUTE Center for Eating Disorders at Denver Health, Denver, Colorado

RICHARD MARTINEZ, MD, MH, DLFAPA
Director of Forensic Psychiatry and Fellowship Training, Robert D. Miller Professor of Forensic Psychiatry, University of Colorado Anschutz Medical Center, Denver, Colorado

MERRILL MATHEW, DO
Attending Psychiatrist, Whiting Forensic Hospital, Middletown, Connecticut

PHILIP MEHLER, MD
Founder and CEO, ACUTE Center for Eating Disorders at Denver Health, Denver, Colorado

LIBBY PARKS, LCSW
Clinical Social Work, ACUTE Center for Eating Disorders at Denver Health, Denver, Colorado

KAILA RUDOLPH, MD, MPH, MBE
Attending Psychiatrist, Department of Consultation-Liaison and Geriatric Psychiatry, Boston Medical Center, Assistant Professor of Psychiatry, Boston University School of Medicine, Department of Psychiatry, Boston, Massachusetts

PATRICIA WESTMORELAND, MD
Medical Director, Women's Unit, The Medical Center of Aurora, Consultant, ACUTE Center for Eating Disorders at Denver Health, Denver, Colorado

JAMES M. WILKINS, MD, DPhil
Medical Director, Cognitive Neuropsychiatry Unit, Division of Geriatric Psychiatry, McLean Hospital, Belmont, Massachusetts, USA; Assistant Professor of Psychiatry, Department of Psychiatry, Harvard Medical School, Boston, Massachusetts

Contents

interdisciplinary models of treatment. The acceptance of SUDs as chronic diseases is essential to expand effective treatments and sustain remission. Creating a culture willing to provide treatment and helping individuals struggling with addiction to accept treatment is the core goal.

This article contextualizes several key ethical issues in consultation-liaison (C-L) psychiatry within historical and principlist frameworks. After summarizing the history of the field, it focuses on 3 main areas of ethical import in C-L psychiatry: decisional capacity assessment, psychosocial evaluations for transplant, and treating mental illness in pregnant patients.

The concept of futility in the treatment of individuals with severe and enduring anorexia nervosa remains controversial and has significant legal and ethical considerations. For those who have been unremittingly ill for 8 to 12 years, full recovery, although possible, is unlikely, and alternatives to traditional, active treatment must be explored. The harm reduction model, palliative care, and end-of-life care are explored as meaningful and reasonable treatments for this population. Landmark cases demonstrating the legal and ethical controversy of such treatment are explored.

Child and adolescent psychiatry involves simultaneously balancing duties to various vulnerable parties. Balancing autonomy and protection for adolescents is complex; state laws governing these situations often add confusion. Common prescribing patterns in child psychiatry lack robust evidence, and utilization of stimulants, atypical antipsychotics, and polypharmacy has skyrocketed. Significant concerns about distributive justice arise from alarming patterns in psychiatric treatment of vulnerable populations, like those affected by poverty, racism, adverse childhood experiences, and certain legal statuses. Principles of justice and respect for persons support the need for safe, adequate, and appropriate psychiatric treatment, including psychosocial interventions and resources, for all children.

Emergency psychiatric practice requires management of both high psychiatric acuity and high ethical complexity. Ethical dilemmas are embedded in the context and practice of agitation management, medical evaluation of uncooperative patients, and involuntary psychiatric hospitalization. Tensions between patient confidentiality and societal interests arise when obtaining collateral information, reporting abuse and neglect, and managing patients who pose a risk of harm toward others. Ultimately, attention to virtue ethics can guide emergency psychiatrists on how to carry out humane and therapeutic care while navigating the ethical principles and legal rules of the emergency psychiatric context.

James M. Wilkins

As dementia progresses and cognitive function declines, surrogate decision making becomes increasingly prevalent. By convention, there is a hierarchical approach to proxy decision making beginning with known wishes, followed by a substituted judgment standard, and then a best-interests standard. For people with dementia, discrepancy in proxy assessments is common and associated with negative behavioral outcomes. Therefore, optimal approaches to proxy decision making for people with dementia should instead prioritize and implement options that encourage direct participation of persons with dementia and standards that explicitly rely on consideration of longitudinal changes in values and preferences for persons with dementia.

PSYCHIATRIC CLINICS OF NORTH AMERICA

FORTHCOMING ISSUES

March 2022
COVID-19: How the Pandemic Changed Psychiatry for Good
Robert L Trestman and Arpan Waghray, *Editors*

June 2022
Workforce and Professional Diversity in Psychiatry
Altha J. Stewart and Howard Y. Liu, *Editors*

RECENT ISSUES

September 2021
Sport Psychiatry: Maximizing Performance
Andy Jagoda and Silvana Riggio, *Editors*

June 2021
Medical Education in Psychiatry
Robert J. Boland and Hermioni L. Amonoo, *Editors*

March 2021
Autism Spectrum Disorder Across the Lifespan Part II
Robert W. Wisner-Carlson, Scott R. Pekrul, Thomas Flis, and Robert Schloesser, *Editors*

SERIES OF RELATED INTEREST

Child and Adolescent Psychiatric Clinics of North America
https://www.childpsych.theclinics.com/

Neurologic Clinics
https://www.neurologic.theclinics.com/

THE CLINICS ARE AVAILABLE ONLINE!
Access your subscription at:
www.theclinics.com

Preface

Psychiatric Ethics in Evolution

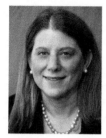 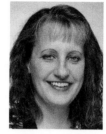

Rebecca Weintraub Brendel, MD, JD   Michelle Hume, MD, PhD

Editors

This issue of *Psychiatric Clinics of North America* was conceived in May of 2019 at the gracious invitation of the series editor, Harsh K. Trivedi, MD, MBA, to whom we are indebted. Amid the collegiality, learning, and intellectual fervor of the American Psychiatric Association (APA) Annual Meeting that year in San Francisco, and in the ensuing months, many of our colleagues on the APA Ethics Committee were delighted to come along on this journey with us by contributing to this exploration of the evolution of psychiatric ethics. When the two of us sat down together, in person, in February of 2020 at the American College of Psychiatrists meeting and finalized the submission invitations and timeline, little did we know that the world as we knew it was about to be upended by the COVID-19 pandemic.

We are indebted to the editorial and production staff at Elsevier for working with us to bring this project to completion amid the substantial disruptions and delays occasioned by the global pandemic. Yet as we reckon with the changes and challenges posed by the pandemic and bring this issue to publication, we have also observed that many of the submissions—conceived prepandemic—have captured essential elements of psychiatric ethics to lead us into the future as we begin to forge the contours of our postpandemic profession.

This issue engages head-on the many ethical challenges ahead for our profession. As psychiatrists and other physicians are increasingly employed by institutions and health care delivery becomes increasingly complex, this ethics compilation begins by interrogating the competing obligations that arise for psychiatrists working in systems of care—often between responsibilities to patients and expectations of institutions. The articles in this issue entitled "Ethical Considerations in Trauma-Informed Care" and "Ethical Challenges in Considerations of Cultural Practices and Traditions: Autonomy and Multiculturalism" squarely return us to the care of the patient with a focus on patient well-being, the patient experience of care, trauma-informed care, and considerations of culture and lived experience.

Psychiatr Clin N Am 44 (2021) xiii–xiv
https://doi.org/10.1016/j.psc.2021.09.001
0193-953X/21/© 2021 Published by Elsevier Inc.   **psych.theclinics.com**

The exploration continues with an unpacking of challenges in psychiatric research, critical to generating knowledge and treatment of mental illness. It next reviews an empirical study of organizational ethics, asking how psychiatry self-regulates in addressing departures from professional norms of ethics and practice. Taken together, these two topics lead us to ask critical questions about our responsibility for generating ethically conducted and scientifically sound research to guide progress in psychiatry in an age of increasing public skepticism about science and about how our profession can meet its responsibility for self-regulation and integrity.

The next seven articles focus attention on emerging ethical challenges across a broad range of psychiatric subspecialty areas and practice. These contributions specifically interrogate ethical challenges in forensic psychiatry, addiction psychiatry, consultation-liaison psychiatry, eating disorders, child and adolescent psychiatry, psychiatric emergencies, and geriatric psychiatry. The careful analysis and wisdom of these articles assure us that, as the cumulative stress, loss, and uncertainty of the COVID-19 pandemic is becoming more fully apparent in our collective psyche, our ethics can help lead the way in addressing the many challenges before us.

Finally, as we bring this project to press, we thank our colleagues for authoring their important contributions to this issue and for their industriousness and commitment to the success of this project amid countless competing obligations of substantial urgency over the past 18 months. We are confident that your work will support countless psychiatrists in never having to worry alone when the inevitable ethical dilemmas arise.

Rebecca Weintraub Brendel, MD, JD
Harvard Medical School Center for Bioethics
641 Huntington Avenue
Second Floor
Boston, MA 02115, USA

Michelle Hume, MD, PhD
Mendota Mental Health Institute
301 Troy Drive
Madison, WI 53704, USA

E-mail addresses:
Rebecca_Brendel@hms.harvard.edu (R.W. Brendel)
Michelle.Hume@dhs.wisconsin.gov (M. Hume)

Ethics in Systems of Care

Charles C. Dike, MD, MPH, FRCPsych[a],*, Merrill Mathew, DO[a],
Amanda Calhoun, MD, MPH[b]

KEYWORDS

- Ethics • Forensic • Systems of care • Managed care • Military ethics • Inpatient
- Multispecialty practice • Pharmaceutical companies

KEY POINTS

As the medical systems of care become increasing complex:

- The traditional and sacred physician-patient relationship loses its simplicity and becomes increasingly nuanced.
- Psychiatrists working in these systems may have divided loyalties to their patients and to their employer that is fraught with potential ethical conflicts.
- Confidentiality, a treating psychiatrist's obligation to keep private their patient's personal or health information without the patient's explicit, informed permission becomes complicated and limited.
- Psychiatrists should be alert to influences or inducements, financial or otherwise, that could impair the primacy of their obligation to patients.
- In working with patients or evaluees, psychiatrists should strive for honesty, objectivity, and informed consent, and be vigilant to situations that could engender bias.

INTRODUCTION

Many psychiatrists work within systems of care, including hospitals, private practice settings, government institutions, accountable care organizations, and others, and often face a multitude of responsibilities to different entities and interests within these roles. Specifically, the sacred fiduciary relationship between a psychiatrist and a patient in treatment itself may engender complicated reactions that often require careful attention of the psychiatrist. When such treatment is provided within the complexity of a system, the psychiatrist's obligations to patients may become even more nuanced and also come into tension with, if not clash with, responsibilities to the institutions and systems in which they increasingly work. These competing obligations, often referred to as "dual agency,"[1] are fraught with ethical conflicts that may be both predictable and unique to the system(s) within which the psychiatrist works.

This article explores ethical dilemmas germane to different systems and settings of care and recommends practical interventions to mitigate or manage them.

[a] L&P Division, CMHC, Yale University School of Medicine, 34 Park Street Rm. 156, New Haven, CT 06519, USA; [b] Yale Child Study Center, 230 S Frontage Road New Haven, CT 06519, USA
* Corresponding author.
E-mail address: Charles.dike@yale.edu

Psychiatr Clin N Am 44 (2021) 507–519
https://doi.org/10.1016/j.psc.2021.08.010
0193-953X/21/© 2021 Elsevier Inc. All rights reserved.

FORENSIC PSYCHIATRIC SETTINGS

"Forensic psychiatry is a subspecialty of psychiatry in which scientific and clinical expertise is applied in legal contexts involving civil, criminal, correctional, regulatory or legislative matters, and in specialized clinical consultations in areas such as risk assessment or employment."[2] Forensic psychiatrists can function in different settings—as a treating psychiatrist in forensic facilities (Department of Correction [DOC] and forensic hospitals), or as a retained consultant to a third party. They may also serve as independent medical examiners to the government or private institutions or companies. In each of these areas, forensic psychiatrists encounter ethical and moral challenges that involve balancing competing interests.

Working in Forensic Institutions

Psychiatrists working directly with patients in a treatment role work within the parameters of the traditional physician-patient relationship to promote the patient's well-being.[1] They may encounter situations, however, where obligations to the patient conflict with responsibilities to the institution or even the public, commonly referred to as dual agency. For example, psychiatrists in forensic institutions are often involved in the assessment and treatment of mentally disordered offenders, including patients admitted for issues related to competency to stand trial, or after a finding of not guilty by reason of insanity (NGRI). Some patients are transfers from DOC for psychiatric stabilization, after which they will return to the DOC. A smaller number of civil patients with severe aggression are sometimes housed in forensic institutions. As a result, the role of the psychiatrist could alternate between treating psychiatrist and forensic evaluator,[3] particularly in smaller systems with limited number of psychiatrists.

As treating physicians, psychiatrists in forensic settings have responsibilities to act in patients' best interests, respecting their choices in accordance with autonomy and promoting their interests and well-being following the ethical principles of beneficence and nonmaleficence. As forensic evaluators, however, psychiatrists' responsibilities to the legal system and the public feature more prominently and while considerations of individual patients cannot be ignored, in forensic evaluative roles, psychiatrists are tasked with serving the interests of justice,[4] thus creating an ethical tension. Forensic evaluations commonly involve gathering and sharing of information, whether favorable or unfavorable, to advance legal proceedings; information obtained from or about the patient may be subject to public scrutiny and individuals may be asked to submit to potentially damaging examination.[3,4] For example, when a treating psychiatrist presents potentially damaging testimony regarding the patient at a hearing to determine the patient's eligibility for community transition, it could interfere with the therapeutic relationship in subsequent encounters, as the patient may question the psychiatrist's motives.[3,4]

To mitigate the effects of competing forensic and clinical duties, one solution is to separate clinical and forensic roles and assign them to different psychiatrists. However, because clinical information is relevant to forensic determinations, potential challenges may remain. In addition, as above, some institutions may not have more than one psychiatrist, making this role separation itself impractical if not impossible. In forensic settings, psychiatrists can advance transparency and ethics by acknowledging their roles and communicating the potential implications to patients. For example, psychiatrists can reinforce and remind a patient of their roles by frequently speaking with the patient about the limits of confidentiality and the implications of the patient's statements and conduct in interactions with the psychiatrist on their legal situation and treatment. Psychiatrists must be careful to describe and clarify their roles, explaining the triangular relationship between themselves, the patient, and the institution. This is also true when patients are on parole, probation, or other supervised (nonhospital) settings. Disclosing this information does not offset the ethical tension, but it shows respect for the patient and provides information to promote informed decision-making by the patient.

Another prominent feature of psychiatrists' role in forensic institutions is the relatively high number of high-risk individuals with significant histories of violence, substance abuse, or antisocial behaviors.[5] Some forensic settings also include a high proportion of sex offenders. Although medication and milieu management along with rehabilitation therapy are important tools of treatment, psychotherapy could pose unique personal and systemic implications for the patient. For example, individual and group therapy sessions that encourage full disclosure of unknown aspects of their history, their current thoughts and plans, and other sources of distress could be detrimental to the patient's release or serve as evidence to prolong custody when documented in forensic reports or presented in court or in front of administrative bodies.[6] Hence, providing effective psychotherapy could present ethical tensions regarding conflicts between treatment roles and forensic settings.

An issue that may be particularly challenging to psychiatrists in forensic settings is the involvement of the criminal legal system in decision-making and oversight regarding treatment options and discharge planning.[5,7] Unlike in regular psychiatric hospitals where a psychiatrist works collaboratively with a patient to develop a treatment plan, requirements set by the judicial system may limit the independence of psychiatrists and the autonomy of the patients in determining the available options. The obligation of the psychiatrist to follow court mandates could raise ethical and practical concerns for the psychiatrist if such mandates are contrary to the psychiatrist's recommended treatment plan or the prevailing community standard of care. Therefore, clear communication between the psychiatrist and the patient about these unique constraints on treatment are imperative. In addition, the psychiatrist also has obligations to the standard of care and the safety of the patient and may find themself in advocacy roles on behalf of the patient, the circumstances of forensic practice, and even to change the very legal system within which they work if the law requires unethical or harmful treatment of persons with mental illness.

Independent Forensic Services

Forensic psychiatrists are involved in evaluations in which they are retained by a third party such as a government or private agency, the judicial system via a private or public attorney, or a private individual. They may be asked to testify in court in civil or criminal cases, in the legislature, or in front of administrative bodies. In these roles, forensic psychiatrists operate outside the medical framework.[8] Here, the essence of the forensic psychiatrist's role is not to promote healing or to relieve suffering, as would be the ethical obligation in treatment settings, but to render a professional opinion that would assist the retaining party in making decisions. Hence, the principle of justice and the obligation to serve social interests may conflict with the principle of beneficence, and nonmaleficence.[8] In their article in this volume, Candilis and Martinez provide a thoughtful engagement of the ethical approaches and paradigms that forensic psychiatrists have engaged in elucidating the contours of ethical responsibility in forensic psychiatry.

Not unlike other forensic settings, the nature of the relationship between the psychiatrist and the evaluee, including confidentiality, emerges once again in this setting. The psychiatrist in the evaluator role must disclose the purpose of the evaluation and their role as evaluator and not treater. This information sharing includes informing the evaluee about whom the psychiatrist is working for and retained by, that they are not functioning in the role of clinical psychiatrist with its confidentiality protections or as the evaluee's psychiatrist, the potential loss of confidentiality, and the potential for the opinion of the psychiatrist to be harmful to the evaluee. A limited physician-patient relationship exists, however,[9] inducing the psychiatrist to be vigilant to risk issues in the evaluee that could warrant immediate care and to respond accordingly. For example, if during an evaluation, the defendant discloses suicidal or homicidal thoughts, the forensic psychiatrist must act to prevent the patient from harming themselves or others.

At the outset of an evaluation for the courts, a forensic psychiatrist can attend to these potentially conflicting and often competing ethical responsibilities through attention to both legal and psychiatric protections and practices. First, for example, forensic evaluees in many if not most circumstances are entitled to seek legal representation and legal advocates may serve to advance the interests of the evaluee in the legal process. Therefore, developing a practice of inquiring about an evaluee's legal representation may advance and/or protect the legal interests and rights of the evaluee. In addition, in accordance with respect for persons, it is the psychiatrist's ethical responsibility to inform the evaluee of the limits on confidentiality and purpose of the evaluation, the terms and nature of the psychiatrist's engagement and the evaluative not treatment nature of the encounter, and any other information relevant to the evaluee's making an informed decision to proceed with the evaluation. Informing the evaluee about how the psychiatrist will communicate the results of the evaluation (report, deposition, testimony, etc.) also advances transparency and the ability to engage in informed consent. Working in the adversarial judicial system of the United States, the psychiatrist should be alert to the risk of conforming opinion to suit the purposes of the retaining party, the evaluee, or the court.[2,10]

The potential for bias or the danger of distorting opinion to benefit the retaining side[2] is an ever-present concern in forensic evaluations. Bias can result from overt or covert pressures such as the desire to please a retaining party to maintain an ongoing financially rewarding relationship or for motives that may be less apparent. Forensic psychiatrists should be open to identifying biases or interests that could influence their opinions in a particular case. For example, a psychiatrist with a history of sexual abuse working as an expert witness on a sex abuse case should explore if the extent of their own lived experience might affect their ability to conduct an objective evaluation. Striving for honesty and objectivity is a central tenet of forensic psychiatric ethics[2] as promulgated by the American Academy of Psychiatry and the Law (AAPL). To mitigate the potential for bias, forensic psychiatrists as a matter of practice make an earnest effort to obtain appropriate collateral information through a comprehensive review of relevant records, interview of important collateral sources, and by requesting relevant investigations such as psychological or neuropsychological evaluations or medical/radiological investigations. Psychiatric examination of the individual is crucial, but may not be possible sometimes, in which case the psychiatrist should state the limitations of the professional opinion rendered as a result. In addition, especially in circumstances in which a forensic psychiatrist is aware of the potential for strong reactions or resonance of a given case with potential implications for the objectivity of the evaluation, seeking peer consultation is an option that can either assist in mitigation of the risk or even the prudence of withdrawing from a case or assignment in extenuating or unforeseen circumstances.

In conclusion, when a psychiatrist's role demands responsibilities to an individual patient or evaluee as well as to a third party such as the legal system, the psychiatrist has assumed a forensic role. This role requires ethical and practice approaches that transcend the traditional physician-patient relationship and routinely requires attention to ethical responsibilities and addressing inherent role tensions. To fulfill the complex and central responsibilities of forensic practice, psychiatrists involved in forensic practice and institutions can manage competing interests and pressures through self-awareness, cultivating skills to identify and address potential and actual ethical tensions and conflicts, and by striving for honesty and objectivity grounded in respect for persons.

HOSPITALS, PRIVATE PRACTICE SETTINGS—GROUP AND MULTISPECIALTY
Inpatient Hospitalization

Psychiatrists working in psychiatric hospitals treat some of the most acutely ill and diagnostically complex psychiatric patients. As such, tensions often run high. Involuntary hospitalization is a constant balance between an individual's autonomy and right to self-determination, care and well-being of the patient, the rights of other patients on the unit and persons outside of the treatment setting who could be exposed to harm as a result of a patient's behavior, and the clinicians' decision-making authority. As such, ethical practice requires psychiatrists to continually balance these interests and reassess the need for involuntary hospitalization on an ongoing basis to advance the least restrictive treatment alternative for the patient. In addition, although the use of force in psychiatric patient care is generally recognized as a necessary practice in certain instances,[11] studies have shown that as many as half of patients admitted involuntarily are unaware of their involuntary status,[12] and that as many as a third of them would have accepted voluntary admission.[12,13] Conversely, as many as half of voluntarily admitted psychiatric patients felt coerced into admission in some way in the hospital.[13,14] These patients' perceptions highlight the importance of honesty and transparency in decision making as a fundamental concern in respecting persons, promoting care (beneficence), avoiding harm (nonmaleficence), and attending to resource allocation and equitable treatment (justice). In addition, coercion has ethical, and in some cases, legal implications.[15]

Another area of potential ethical tension may occur when psychiatrists work on multidisciplinary hospital teams, often composed of residents, nurses, psychologists, social workers, rehabilitation therapists, peer support specialists, and patient advocates, among others. Psychiatrists may feel pressured by the opinions of other members on the team to provide certain types of care, take away or restrict patient privileges, or place a patient in restraints or seclusion. When patients perceive that they are treated with respect and dignity and that their opinion in their care is taken seriously, it enhances therapeutic alliance and decreases maladaptive behaviors such as violence.[16] It is psychiatrists' ethical responsibility to put patient interests first and where these interests come into tension with other competing interests, ensure that they are nonetheless considered prominently.[1]

Private Practice Settings

Ethical tensions are not limited to public institutional settings. In an era of ever more complex practice arrangements, competing responsibilities may also occur in private practice settings. For example, a private practice group could be single specialty and limited to psychiatrists or multispecialty including physicians from different areas of medicine. Practice groups may also include members from different professional backgrounds and levels of licensure. For example, a mental health practice group might include psychiatrists alongside psychologists, social workers (as therapists or case managers), licensed professional counselors, nurses, addiction counselors, or any combination of disciplines. Ethics guidance and practice regarding the management of patients could vary in key features depending on training, professional licensure, and disciplinary background. For example, although American Psychiatric Association (APA) Principles of Medical Ethics prohibit sexual relationships with any current or former patient,[17] it is permissible for physicians from other specialties and psychologists to become romantically involved with former patients (and family members of patients) under certain circumstances.[18] Although group practice settings present opportunities for better coordination of care between disciplines and specialties, "they also create potential for conflict between the primacy of the individual patient and the legal, business and political interests of the care system of which the psychiatrist should be aware and monitor."[1] It is important for psychiatrists, therefore, to be aware of key areas of potential discordance in ethics guidance to create consistent expectations and standards for care of patients in private practices in which they have oversight, supervisory, and business interests.

Specifically, in group practices, the roles and responsibilities of the various treatment team members should be clearly defined as ethical tensions can arise regarding responsibility for decisions. When collaborating with other professionals in a mental health practice, although responsibility for the overall treatment of a patient is shared, the responsibility often weighs more heavily toward the psychiatrist, especially regarding medications and medical matters[18].

Psychiatrists should also be aware that business practices and financial interest of group practices may come into tension with responsibilities to patients as well as with regulatory and legal requirements for group practices.[19] In particular, psychiatrists should avoid the practice and/or appearance of fee-splitting and remuneration for referrals,[20] incentives to overtreat or provide care that is not medically necessary, and refrain from providing care for profit motives. Referrals of patients within group practices should advance the care of the patient, not occur for the purpose of benefitting the referring psychiatrist or the psychiatrist's practice. Referral of patients to therapists or other practitioners employed by the psychiatrist may occur if it advances the competent care of the patient.

Attention to patient-centered care equally applies when decisions about services provided to patients are made at levels above the authority of a psychiatrist hired by a group practice. For example, if a nonphysician director of a private practice group makes treatment decisions or dictates treatment practices that place cost-cutting or financial remuneration above patient care, the psychiatrist has an ethical obligation to resist these decisions, and to advocate for organizational ethics supportive of patient care. Likewise, psychiatrists should not feel pressured to sign off on treatment plans which in their opinion, are not in the patients' best interest, understanding that as licensed physicians, responsibility for treatment ultimately rests with them both ethically and legally.

In group practice settings, a psychiatrist's responsibility to address impaired, dangerous, or ethically suspect conduct of colleagues may also arise. Some situations occasioning a responsibility to act might include substance use[21] or a boundary crossing or violation such as an inappropriate personal relationship with a patient.[22] Confronting colleagues is not only uncomfortable, but it can be contentious and has the potential to strain the collegiality of a group practice and damage professional relationships. However, ignoring unethical behavior is not an option. Addressing the behavior does not necessarily mean reporting to the licensing board or ethics committee. Ethics guidance calls for a response by the colleague, and several options are available to begin to address concerns about colleagues' practice.[22] An initial attempt might include a resolution through informal and more collegial means, but if it fails, reporting upward through appropriate channels of authority to ensure the protection of patients. If all efforts fail or if a patient is in immediate danger, then a report to licensing authority may be warranted.[1]

SYSTEMS AND ORGANIZATIONS: MANAGED CARE, DRUG COMPANIES, AND THE MILITARY AND GOVERNMENT
Managed Care Organizations

With the ever-complex reimbursement structure and review of mental health payment, psychiatrists fill various roles in managed care organizations (MCOs) including in utilization review, consultation to disability analysts, or rendering independent medical evaluations.[23] In all these roles, the psychiatrists do not have a treating relationship with patients but rather perform work for the company that hired them. Despite the view of some psychiatrists that working for MCO is tantamount to working for the "dark side",[24] there are some clear benefits for psychiatrists to serve in these roles compared with nonpsychiatrists. Not only do psychiatrists speak the same language and have the ability to understand the challenges of treating psychiatrists seeking care for patients, their experience as clinicians will also help in the decision-making process of approval or denial of services.[25]

However, ethical tensions arise for psychiatrists working as utilization reviewers for MCOs, chief of which involves questions of the primacy of obligations. Specifically, do psychiatrists in systems of care owe their responsibilities to patients or the MCOs? The Hippocratic Oath,[26] AMA's Code of Medical Ethics,[27] and APA Principles of Medical Ethics[28] all emphasize the primacy of patient well-being as the core ethical obligations of all physicians, including psychiatrists. Central to the analysis of the ethical moorings of physician conduct in performing utilization review (UR) for MCOs and other organizations is the question of what activities qualify as the practice of medicine. For example, psychiatrist-utilization reviewers must hold a license to practice medicine to be eligible for hire, and they make decisions based on their medical education, training, knowledge, and expertise. Hence, it would be reasonable to simply say that UR constitutes the practice of medicine. As a legal matter, courts have varied in their rulings regarding this issue. For example, the Arizona court of appeals ruled in 1997[29] that physicians involved in UR activities are in fact, practicing medicine as decisions require the use of professional and clinical judgment.[29] In contrast, other courts have reached a different conclusion, that UR is not the practice of medicine,[30,31] or it could be the practice of medicine depending on the specifics of the individual case,[32] thereby necessitating a case-by-case analysis to make the determination. From the professional and organizational ethics perspective, the APA ethics committee in 2015 specifically addressed questions about psychiatrists' roles in UR to address questions from members.[21] Based on the fact that the psychiatrist utilization reviewer is not a treating psychiatrist, the committee opined that "...the psychiatrist managed care or utilization reviewer owes his primary obligation to the managed care company and a secondary one to the patient...it is not the ethics responsibility of the reviewing psychiatrist to determine whether the plan is meeting parity law requirements....the primary duty of the reviewing psychiatrist in this situation is to evaluate whether the requested treatment is warranted and covered by the plan."[21] This guidance, however, emphasized that patient interests and responsibility of psychiatrists to patients cannot be discounted; indeed, psychiatrists working in MCOs cannot wholly ignore the needs of patients and should continue to advocate for changes in the managed care plan that would benefit patients.

Pharmaceutical Companies

In recent years, the relationship between psychiatrists and pharmaceutical companies has come under public scrutiny. For example, in 2018, PsychCentral published the names of the top 50 psychiatrists[33] who had earned more than $100,000 from pharmaceutical companies (PCs) between 2009 and 2010, raising questions of objectivity and ethics. Increasing concerns of the problematic relationship between physicians and pharmaceutical companies prompted Senators Chuck Grassley and Herb Kohl to introduce the Physician Sunshine Payment Act, first in 2007, when it failed to pass, and consistently thereafter until 2009 when it passed into law.[34] Act II of the Sunshine Act, or the Sunshine Act's Final Rule,[35] was passed into law in 2013. The law requires drug, device, and biologic makers to report annually, payments to doctors to the Department of Health and Human Services and to publish those payments online for public information.

Although the relationship between psychiatrists and PCs is not new, recent understanding of the deleterious influence of PCs on most areas of medical practice has had a negative impact on psychiatry as a profession, and on individual psychiatrists.[36] In his 2013 book, Saving Normal,[37] Allen Francis, a professor of psychiatry and chair of the APA's task force overseeing the revision of (DSM-IV), warned of Big Pharma's influence in overdiagnosis of psychiatric disorders, overmedicalization of normal behavior and intense advocacy for prescription of medications to manage them. Dr Francis voiced the concern already reflected in literature[38] regarding the financial ties between the developers of the DSM and the pharmaceutical industry. In addition, the report that 60% of medical school department chairs receive personal income from PCs, most often as a consultant or member of a scientific advisory board[36] and that over 60% of experts involved in the development of DSM 5 had ties to PCs[39] is particularly troubling. In response, the APA has laid out a comprehensive Project Specific Conflict of Interest (COI) policy[40] "...to ensure the highest level of ethical standards in activities entered on behalf of the APA and American Psychiatric Association Foundation (APAF) as it relates to promoting objectivity in research. The expectation is that the design, conduct, and reporting of grants, contracts, and cooperative agreements are free from bias due to any potential or perceived conflict of financial interest as well as to ensure the APA/APAF compliance with federal, state, local, and institutional policies.[40]" Furthermore, "the APA has adopted a policy of maximum disclosure of Participant's Affiliations and Interests from anyone participating in its governance and component structure. Such disclosure is necessary to ensure the integrity of the APA's policies, positions, publications and other services and to protect the Participants, the APA and the profession.[41]"

That said, the relationship between psychiatrists and PCs is not always negative. PCs have supported educational programs and research, as well as sponsored scientific conferences. It is, however, at these different levels of interaction that ethical conflicts are likely to emerge. Research shows that doctors are more likely to prescribe medications promoted by pharmaceutical representatives from whom they have received gifts.[42] Also, researchers sponsored by PCs are more likely to minimize adverse effects of the medications in development and to enhance positive results while downplaying negative ones.[43] Furthermore, paid psychiatric consultants and speakers are more likely to induce their colleagues through strong advocacy, to prescribe medications off-label for indications without proven research as the case of gabapentin illustrates as a prime example.[44] Of particular concern is the influence of PCs on the development of clinical practice guidelines directing the use of certain medications made by the sponsoring PCs.[45] As a result, pharmaceutical companies expend significant financial resources to court physicians/psychiatrists. For example, companies have flown doctors on business class tickets to foreign conferences, housed them and dined them in choice hotels, and given them expensive tickets to sporting events, cruises, and other perks.[46] These sponsorship activities may hurt patients in a variety of ways; from decreasing access to medications due to exorbitant prices, to influencing research findings that minimize or exclude serious adverse effects, to influencing prescribing practices that may not be in the best interest of patients. Finally, even the appearance of financial conflict-of-interest may damage the reputation of psychiatrists, leads to loss of trust for the profession, and ultimately discourages help seeking by those who need it most.

To protect patients, psychiatrists may respond in a variety of ways.[43] For example, psychiatrists and organizations may decrease direct influence by declining gifts and perks from PCs, learning to critically analyze data for themselves, refusing direct funding for individual researchers but not of research in general, declining sponsorship of conferences and educational activities that promote medications from sponsors, and publicly stating their conflicts of interest—actual and potential. In addition, PCs should publish, on a regular basis, expenditures made to physicians, medical organizations and universities. As noted earlier, these payments are now subject to congressional and public scrutiny as required by the Sunshine Act.[35]

Military and Government Systems

Military psychiatrists may encounter ethical tensions in their practice when medical and psychiatric ethics come into conflict with military responsibilities and the Uniformed Code of Military Justice. In addition, there is pressure to abide by the mission of military medical officer to "maintain the fighting force."[47] In other words, as military officers, military psychiatrists have responsibilities to the armed services, maintaining the force, and to the country yet as psychiatrists they have obligations to patients. One need not look too far into the responsibilities of a military psychiatrist to encounter frequent ethical challenges. For example, the confidentiality of individual patients—who are also service members—brings dual loyalty to the forefront: by maintaining the confidentiality of a patient, the psychiatrist could be putting other service members at risk or risking national security in a sensitive operation. Other professional activities such as fitness for duty or deployment, disability and separation from service evaluations are also complicated by the fact that military interests and the individual interests of a service member-patient can be at odds. As in all competing loyalty situations, military psychiatrists can manage the tensions with truthfulness about the limits of confidentiality of evaluations and treatment, including highlighting situations in which the commanding officer or other parties may have access to their health information. Awareness of the limits of confidentiality enhances informed consent by providing information of relevance to decisions about evaluation and treatment. Deployment and operational constraints may additionally require disclosures about limitations in available treatments and services at the location of deployment.[47] Informed consent is also promoted by discussion of potential consequences of psychiatric treatment to the patient's career.[47]

Another important ethical consideration in military psychiatry is the maintenance of boundaries. The tight-knit community of military bases and operations as well as the limited number of psychiatrists result in situations in which the psychiatrist is responsible for the care of friends and companions, as well as junior or senior officers, creating the possibility and actuality of boundary crossings and violations. In anticipation of the unique and varied nature of military operations and functions, the psychiatrist may advance ethical care by establishing ground rules and expectations at the outset of the treatment or other evaluation and share ways that potential conflicts that arise in the future will be managed.[47]

The issue of participation in interrogations became prominent during the war on terror. In recent years, both the APA[48] and AMA[49] have laid out ethics principles regarding the interrogation of detainees. Similar to the AMA's ethics opinion, the APA[48] states that: "psychiatrists should not participate in, or otherwise assist or facilitate, commission of torture of any person; ...No psychiatrist should participate directly in the interrogation of persons held in custody by military or civilian investigative or law enforcement authorities, whether in the United States or elsewhere." Direct participation was broadly defined. Psychiatrists could, however, "provide training to military or civilian investigative or law enforcement personnel on recognizing and responding to persons with mental illnesses, on the possible medical and psychological effects of particular techniques and conditions of interrogation, and on other areas within their professional expertise." Psychiatrists providing direct medical care to detainees have a physician-patient relationship with the detainees with limits as stated earlier. Though there are limits to confidentiality in the public interest, as for any treatment, these limits may be more extensive where national security is concerned.

SUMMARY

In conclusion, given the many settings and systems of care in which psychiatrists serve both clinical and nonclinical roles, psychiatrists can expect to increasingly encounter ethical tensions and even conflicts between responsibilities to systems and institutions and to patients and persons. Through careful and attuned awareness, honesty, and transparency, psychiatrists may reduce and even resolve these conflicts. Attention to core tenets of medical and psychiatric ethics and awareness of resources to address these conflicts can advance the ethical conduct of psychiatrists. Psychiatrists have responsibilities to develop contextual and systems awareness to inform their practice and conduct.

TAKE-HOME POINTS

As the medical systems of care become increasing complex:
- The traditional and sacred physician-patient relationship loses its simplicity and becomes increasingly nuanced.
- Psychiatrists working in these systems may have divided loyalties, to their patients and to their employer, a dual role or dual agency that cannot be avoided in certain circumstances but is fraught with potential ethical conflicts.
- Confidentiality, a treating psychiatrist's obligation to keep private their patient's personal or health information without the patient's explicit, informed permission becomes complicated and limited.
- For a patient's consent to care to be truly informed, the limits of confidentiality and the limitations on the care provided must be comprehensively discussed and understood.
- Psychiatrists should be alert to influences or inducements, financial or otherwise, that could impair the primacy of their obligation to patients.
- In working with patients or evaluees, psychiatrists should strive for honesty and objectivity, and be vigilant to situations that could engender bias.
- A psychiatrist's loyalty to a third party does not include participation in torture or interrogation of detainees.

REFERENCES

1. Brendel RW, Dike CC, Ginzburg H, et al. American Psychiatric Association Commentary on Ethics in Practice 2015. Available at: https://www.psychiatry.org/File%20Library/Psychiatrists/Practice/Ethics/APA-Commentary-on-Ethics-in-Practice.pdf. Accessed August 27, 2021.

2. American Academy of Psychiatry and the Law: Ethical Guidelines for the Practice of Forensic Psychiatry. 2005. Available at: https://www.aapl.org/ethics.htm. Accessed June 4, 2020.

3. Cervantes AN, Hanson A. Dual agency and ethics conflicts in correctional practice: sources and solutions. J Am Acad Psychiatry Law 2013;41(1):72–8.

4. Niveau G, Welle I. Forensic psychiatry, one subspecialty with two ethics? A systematic review. BMC Med Ethics 2018;19(1):25.

5. Norko M, Dike CC. In: Sharfstein SS, Dickerson FB, Oldham JM, editors. The forensic unit. Textbook of hospital psychiatry. Washington, DC: American Psychiatric Publishing Inc.; 2008. p. 185–95.

6. Kersting K. New hope for sex offender treatment. Monitor Psychol 2003;34(7):52. Available at: https://www.apa.org/monitor/julaug03/newhope. Accessed September 30, 2021.

7. Kapoor R, Dike C, Norko MA. Psychiatric treatment in forensic hospital and correctional settings. Psychiatr Ann 2018;48(2):102–8.

8. Appelbaum PS. The parable of the forensic psychiatrist: ethics and the problem of doing harm. Int J Law Psychiatry 1990;13:249–59.

9. American Medical Association: AMA Code of medical ethics, opinion 1.2.6 work-related and independent medical examinations. Chicago (IL): AMA. Available at: https://www.ama-assn.org/delivering-care/ethics/work-related-independent-medical-examinations. Accessed August 27, 2021.

10. Gold LH, Anfang SA, Drukteinis AM, et al. AAPL practice guideline for the forensic evaluation of psychiatric disability. J Am Acad Psychiatry Law 2008; 36:S3–50.

11. Høyer G. On the justification for civil commitment. Acta Psychiatr Scand Suppl 2000;101:65–71.

12. Monahan J, Hoge S, Lidz C, et al. Coercion and commitment: Understanding involuntary mental hospital admission. Int J Law Psychiatry 1995;18:249–63.

13. Iversen KI, Høyer G, Sexton H, et al. Perceived coercion among patients admitted to acute wards in Norway. Nord J Psychiatry 2002;56:433–9.

14. Brakel SJ, Parry J, Weiner B. The mentally disabled and the law. American Bar Foundation, Chicago (IL)

15. Wynn DR. Coercion in psychiatric care: clinical, legal, and ethical controversies. Int J Psychiatry Clin Pract 2006;10(4):247–51.

16. Dike CC. In: Griffith EEH, Norko MA, Buchanan A, et al, editors. Management of forensic hospitals: bearing witness to change in forensic psychiatry and psychology practice. Boca Raton (FL): CRC Press; 2016. p. 219–33.

17. American Psychiatric Association. The Principles of Medical Ethics With Annotations Especially Applicable to Psychiatry. 2013. Available at: https://www.psychiatry.org/psychiatrists/practice/ethics. Accessed August 27, 2021.

18. American Medical Association Code of Medical Ethics 9.1.1. Romantic or Sexual Relationship with Patients. Available at: https://www.ama-assn.org/delivering-care/ethics/romantic-or-sexual-relationships-patients. Accessed September 30, 2021.

19. Brendel RW, Dike CC, Ginzburg H, et al. American Psychiatric Association Commentary on Ethics in Practice 2015; Topic 3.3.2. Available at: https://www.psychiatry.org/psychiatrists/practice/ethics. Accessed August 27, 2021.

20. Brendel RW, Dike CC, Ginzburg H, et al. American Psychiatric Association Commentary on Ethics in Practice 2015; Topic 3.4.1. Available at: https://www.psychiatry.org/psychiatrists/practice/ethics. Accessed August 27, 2021.

21. Brendel RW, Dike CC, Ginzburg H, et al. American Psychiatric Association Commentary on Ethics in Practice 2015; Topic 3.3.4. Available at: https://www.psychiatry.org/psychiatrists/practice/ethics. Accessed August 27, 2021.

22. American Psychiatric Association: Opinions of the Ethics Committee on the Principles of Medical Ethics With Annotations Especially Applicable to Psychiatry 2015. Available at: https://www.psychiatry.org/psychiatrists/practice/ethics. Accessed June 4, 2020.

23. Brendel RW, Dike CC, Ginzburg H, et al. American Psychiatric Association Commentary on Ethics in Practice 2015; Topic 3.3.5. Available at: https://www.psychiatry.org/psychiatrists/practice/ethics. Accessed August 27, 2021.

24. Careers for Physicians in Managed Care and Utilization Management. 2021. Available at: https://lookforzebras.com/nonclinical-careers-utilization-management/. Accessed August 27, 2021.

25. Buttz L. Working for insurers: a view from the dark side. Family practice management. Available at: https://www.aafp.org/fpm/2008/0700/p19.pdf. Accessed June 8, 2020.

26. Moawad H. Succeeding as a Utilization Reviewer. HCPLive 2019. Available at: https://www.hcplive.com/view/succeeding-as-a-physician-in-utilization-review. Accessed August 27, 2021.

27. Miles SH. The hippocratic Oath and the ethics of medicine. New York: Oxford University Press; 2004.

28. American Medical Association Code of Medical Ethics: Patient-Physician Relationship. Available at: https://www.ama-assn.org/delivering-care/ethics/code-medical-ethics-patient-physician-relationships. Accessed June 8, 2020.

29. Murphy v Board of Medical Examiners of the State of Arizona, 949 P. 2d 530 (Ariz. Ct. App. 1997). Available at: https://caselaw.findlaw.com/az-court-of-appeals/1134683.html. Accessed September 30, 2021.

30. 1999-044 Ohio Attorney General Opinions. OAG 99-044. Available at: https://www.ohioattorneygeneral.gov/getattachment/8c6bc3d9-bb34-406f-aece-4231c6c30f03/1999-044.aspx. Accessed June 9, 2020.

31. Scott RL. Are Medical Directors Performing Utilization Review "Practicing Medicine"? 1999. Available at: https://www.law.uh.edu/healthlaw/perspectives/MedicalProfessionals/991014Are.html. Accessed June 9, 2020.

32. Morris v. District of Columbia Board of Medicine, 701 A. 2d 364 (D.C. 1997). New York: Available at: http://oag.dc.gov/sites/default/files/2018-02/Opinion-July-2014-License-to-Practice.pdf. Accessed September 30, 2021.

33. Grohol JM. Top 50 Psychiatrists Paid by Insurance Companies. Available at: https://psychcentral.com/blog/top-50-psychiatrists-paid-by-pharmaceutical-companies/. Accessed June 8, 2020.

34. Library of Congress. Bill Summary and Status, 111th Congress (2009–2010). S. 301 – Physician Payments Sunshine Act of 2009. 2009. Available at: https://www.congress.gov/bill/111th-congress/senate-bill/301/text. Accessed August 27, 2021.

35. Pham-Kanter G. Act II of the Sunshine Act. PLoS Med 2014;11(11):e1001754.

36. Insel TR. Psychiatrists' relationships with pharmaceutical companies: part of the problem or part of the solution? JAMA 2010;303(12):1192–3.

37. Frances A. Saving normal: an insider's revolt against out-of-control psychiatric diagnosis, DSM-5, Big Pharma, and the medicalization of ordinary life. New York: William Morrow & Co; 2013.

38. Cosgrove L, Krimsky S, Vijayaraghavan M, et al. Financial ties between DSM-IV panel members and the pharmaceutical industry. Psychother Psychosom 2006; 75(3):154–60.

39. Cosgrove L, Bursztajn H, Krimsky S. Developing unbiased diagnostic and treatment guidelines in psychiatry. N Engl J Med 2009;360:2035–6.

40. American Psychiatric Association and American Psychiatric Association Foundation Project Specific Conflict of Interest Policy: Per 42 CFR Part 50 Subpart F. Available at: https://www.psychiatry.org/conflict-of-interest-policy. Accessed August 27, 2021.

41. American Psychiatric Association Disclosure of Interest Policy. 2020. Available at: https://www.psychiatry.org/File%20Library/About-APA/Organization-Documents-Policies/apa-discolsure-of-interests-policy.pdf. Accessed August 27, 2021.

42. Fickweiler F, Fickweiler W, Urbach E. Interactions between physicians and the pharmaceutical industry generally and sales representatives specifically and their association with physicians' attitudes and prescribing habits: a systematic review. BMJ Open 2017;7(9):e016408.

43. Green S. Ethics and the Pharmaceutical Industry. Australas Psychiatry 2008; 16(3):158–65.

44. Kassirer J. On the take: how America's complicity with big business can endanger your health. New York: Oxford Press; 2005.

45. Cosgrove L, Bursztajn HJ, Krimsky S, et al. Conflicts of interest and disclosure in the American Psychiatric Association's Clinical Practice Guidelines. Psychother Psychosom 2009;78(4):228–32.

46. Boseley S, Evans R. Drug Giants accused over Doctor's Perks. Guardian Newspaper. 2008. Available at: https://www.theguardian.com/society/2008/aug/23/health.pharmaceuticals. Accessed June 8, 2020.

47. Wagner CH, Appenzeller GN, Grieger TA, et al. Ethical considerations in military psychiatry. Psychiatr Clin North Am 2009;32(2):271–81.

48. Position Statement on psychiatric participation in interrogation of detainees. Available at: https://www.psychiatry.org/file%20library/about-apa/organization-documents-policies/policies/position-psychiatric-participation-in-interrogation-of-detainees.pdf. Accessed August 27, 2021.

49. Physician Participation in Interrogation: AMA Code of Ethics Opinion 9.7.4. Available at: https://www.ama-assn.org/delivering-care/ethics/physician-participation-interrogation. Accessed August 27, 2021.

Ethical Considerations in Trauma-Informed Care

Kaila Rudolph, MD, MPH, MBE[a,b,*]

KEYWORDS

- Clinical ethics • Trauma-informed care • PTSD

KEY POINTS

- Trauma-Informed Care (TIC) is grounded in the understanding that exposure to trauma is common and can have significant impact on patient health, care engagement, and provider well-being.
- TIC strategies in health care settings aim to support the needs of trauma survivors and facilitate their safety and participation in care.
- TIC approaches prioritize staff training and education to promote safety, trustworthiness and transparency, and empowerment and collaborative care decision making, with routine screening for trauma exposure and linkage to appropriate mental health care services.
- Implementation of TIC approaches are supported by feminist, narrative, and principlist ethical frameworks and require a multilevel approach spanning legislative, organizational, and provider-level interventions to be successful.

ETHICAL CONSIDERATIONS IN TRAUMA-INFORMED CARE
Defining Trauma

Lifetime exposure to a traumatic event is common.[1] A large population-based survey of 68,894 adults across 24 countries and 6 continents, including the United States, demonstrated that 70.4% of participants experienced at least 1 traumatic event, with 30.5% experiencing more than 4 traumatic events in their lifetime.[1] Despite the widespread global prevalence of trauma, defining trauma and traumatic effects and identifying and reducing their impact on mental and physical health remains challenging.[2]

The Substance Abuse and Mental Health Services Administration (SAMHSA) defines individual trauma as "An event, series of events, or set of circumstances that is experienced by an individual as physically or emotionally harmful or life-threatening and that has lasting adverse effects on the individual's functioning and

[a] Department of Consultation-Liaison and Geriatric Psychiatry, Boston Medical Center, Doctor's Office Building, 720 Harrison Avenue, Suite 7600, Boston, MA 02118, USA; [b] Department of Psychiatry, Boston University School of Medicine, Boston, MA, USA
* Department of Consultation-Liaison and Geriatric Psychiatry, Boston Medical Center, Doctor's Office Building, 720 Harrison Avenue, Suite 7600, Boston, MA 02118.
E-mail address: Kaila.Rudolph@bmc.org

Psychiatr Clin N Am 44 (2021) 521–535
https://doi.org/10.1016/j.psc.2021.07.001
0193-953X/21/© 2021 Elsevier Inc. All rights reserved.

psych.theclinics.com

mental, physical, social, emotional, or spiritual well-being."[3] The Diagnostic and Statistical Manual, Fifth Edition (DSM-5) highlights that traumatic events may involve direct experience, witnessing an event occurring to others, learning of a traumatic event impacting loved ones, or repeated/extreme exposure to distressing components of a traumatic event.[4] SAMHSA identifies 3 core components to the definition of trauma: the occurrence of a traumatic event, the person's experience of this event, and the long-lasting adverse effects that occur following the event and experience.[3] SAMHSA's approach highlights the common understanding of trauma as a process involving the interaction of the traumatic event(s) and individual experience, with vulnerability and resilience factors that may change over time.[5] Beyond individual trauma, traumatic experiences may occur at the community, cultural, or population level, with historical trauma referring to group traumatic experiences persisting via dissemination across generations within a community.[5]

Traumatic events may encompass a diverse array of potential exposures across the life span. The DSM-5 highlights individual-level exposures of "actual or threatened death, serious injury, and sexual violence."[4] Individual traumas typically occur within the context of a community, with community-level traumas including environmental disasters, war, and structural violence or discrimination.[3] Globally, the most common forms of traumatic events have been identified as accidents or injuries, witnessing death or serious injury, and robbery.[1] Trauma exposure is associated with physical and mental health adverse effects.[2]

The Impact of Trauma on Health

Health behaviors, such as diet and exercise, exert a significant impact on risk of morbidity and mortality.[6] Limited engagement in health-promoting behaviors has been linked to trauma exposure.[7] The Adverse Childhood Experiences (ACE) study by Felitti and colleagues[7] retrospectively surveyed 9508 adults, who had undergone a standardized medical evaluation, about their experience of childhood adverse events, including physical or sexual abuse and exposure to household dysfunction. A significant association was found between exposure to childhood adversity and engagement in high-risk health behaviors, such as smoking, inactivity, high-risk sexual behavior, substance use, and suicide attempt.[7] Similarly, childhood trauma exposure was significantly associated with adulthood medical conditions, including cancer, ischemic heart disease, chronic obstructive pulmonary disease, and self-rated poor health.[7] Exposure to childhood trauma has also been shown to affect the stress response and affect regulation through alterations in the hypothalamic-pituitary-adrenal axis causing cortisol dysregulation, and disruption in development of the hippocampus and frontal-limbic systems contributing to dysfunction of regulatory neural systems.[8] Trauma exposure is also linked to the development of mental health conditions such as posttraumatic stress disorder (PTSD), mood disorders, and substance use disorders.[9] Finally, trauma exposure has been conceptualized as cumulative, with the greater the trauma exposure, the greater the impact on physical and mental health.[10]

Persons with mental illness are at even greater risk of trauma exposure than the general population.[11] For example, in a sample of 142 persons with severe, persistent mental illness and past history of psychiatric hospitalization, trauma exposure rates were found to be as high as 87% for experiencing 1 trauma event and 58% for personally experiencing either physical or sexual assault.[11] Consistent with this high occurrence of trauma exposure, the prevalence of PTSD in this patient study population was 30% using DSM-based criteria, aligning with existing literature supporting higher rates of PTSD in persons with mental health concerns than in the general population.[9,11] Existing research also highlights the complex interplay between trauma exposure, PTSD, and comorbid depression, substance use, and mental and physical health status.[9] Specifically, increased trauma exposure is associated with higher severity PTSD, which is, in turn, associated with more severe depression and reduced overall mental and physical health.[9] The negative health effects of PTSD are also linked to economic impact, with associated work impairment and an estimated lifetime cost of childhood interpersonal violence exposure at more than $55 billion nationwide.[12]

Mental health conditions are a risk factor for trauma, and paradoxically, mental health treatment has also been associated with retraumatization, when a present experience serves as a reminder for a past traumatic event.[10] Practices such as restraints, seclusion, and forced medication administration, which may occur in medical, mental health, and emergency settings, have been linked to harmful effects for patients who witness and personally experience these interventions as well as for health care providers.[10] In addition to traumatizing health care exposures, past trauma exposure has been linked to reduced engagement with clinical care, which may further contribute to worsened health.[13] Trauma exposures may predispose persons to experience care as distressing and traumatic, with mistrust and avoidance of clinical care, creating barriers to care engagement.[13] Trauma is therefore both a risk factor for the development of health challenges and may pose challenges for engagement with care to address these health comorbidities.[13]

In additional to mental health conditions, it is important to note the existence of racial and ethnic disparities in trauma exposure. Higher rates of child mistreatment and exposure to interpersonal violence have been noted in Black and Hispanic persons, with higher rates of PTSD among Black persons compared with non-Hispanic White persons. Despite higher rates of PTSD, members of minority racial and ethnic groups have been found to be less likely to receive mental health treatment for PTSD, a finding consistent with existing racial and ethnic health and care access disparities.[14] Broadly considering the impact of additional social determinants of health, such as poverty and homelessness, is important because these factors are also associated with increased trauma exposure.[15,16]

Clinical Vignette

While on call in your hospital's psychiatric emergency department, you receive a page from an emergency medicine colleague concerning Ms E, a 27-year-old woman, with a psychiatric history significant for borderline personality disorder. She has a past history of self-harm gestures, with 1 suicide attempt via overdose, for which she was psychiatrically hospitalized when she was 15 years old. She has an outpatient psychiatrist and is not prescribed psychotropic pharmacotherapy. She has no significant past medical history. You inquire about any known trauma history. The emergency physician informs you that she did not feel comfortable obtaining a trauma history. You discuss the importance of screening all patients for past trauma, given the impact of trauma on their experience and engagement with care, especially in emergency settings that can be retraumatizing.

Ms E presented to the emergency department following vaginal foreign body insertion, a tampon inserted more than 48 hours prior. She refused to remove the tampon, leading her mother to bring her to the emergency room for further evaluation and care. At this time, Ms E is medically stable, although she has developed a low-grade fever and mild white blood cell count elevation concerning for the potential development of toxic shock syndrome. Ms E declined pelvic examination and foreign body removal. The consultation question you receive is for capacity to refuse removal of the foreign body.

TRAUMA-INFORMED CARE: RATIONALE AND CORE PRINCIPLES

Widespread trauma exposure, globally and within the United States, combined with evidence that trauma is associated with poor health and high health care costs, has contributed to a shift from a biomedical care paradigm centered on disease process and treatment to one that includes emphasizing attunement to psychosocial factors and the impact of trauma on health.[8] Trauma-informed care (TIC) has been defined as "a strengths-based framework that is grounded in an understanding of and responsiveness to the impact of trauma, that emphasizes physical, psychological, and emotional safety for both providers and survivors, and that creates opportunities for survivors to rebuild a sense of control and empowerment."[8] TIC is not aimed at directly managing symptoms of trauma and does not require expertise in trauma mental health treatment, but rather can be universally implemented for all patients in a care setting.[8] Instead, TIC recognizes that effective treatment occurs in the context of a patient's life history and lived experience, and is most effective when structured and delivered to ensure safety and patient empowerment. TIC also recognizes the potential trauma to clinical staff from their professional roles, especially in high-acuity and high-risk situations. TIC contrasts trauma-specific care, which aims to treat clinical symptoms that have developed from trauma and requires trauma-care expertise.[8]

TIC is based on 4 core assumptions: (1) trauma impacts health and clinical care; (2) trauma screening must be completed with provision of appropriate care services; (3) TIC can assist providers in responding to the widespread presence of trauma; and (4) retraumatization may be reduced through adaptation of care/organizational practices to reduce triggering of traumatic memories and further traumatization.[3] TIC may be applied across all levels of health care, from the individual patient to the institutional level, where hospital policy implementation may promote TIC education and training.[3,8]

SAMHSA identifies 6 core principles that are central to implementation of a TIC approach[3]: (1) Safety: Staff and patients should have an experience of physical and psychological safety within the clinical environment and in their interpersonal interactions; (2) Trustworthiness and transparency: Decisions and policies made within the health care setting are clearly communicated to staff and patients to promote trust and collaborative decision making; (3) Peer support: Individuals with lived experience of trauma may be consulted to provide guidance and support to patients to promote their recovery; (4) Collaboration and mutuality: Promotion of partnerships, with minimization of power differentials between staff and patients, and recognition that everyone plays a role in TIC; (5) Empowerment, voice, and choice: Recognition of the strengths of patients to foster shared decision making, goal setting, resilience, and hope of healing from trauma; and (6) Cultural, historical, and gender issues: The implementation of programs and policies that are responsive to the cultural, gender, and racial needs of the patients and staff served.[3]

In summary, a TIC approach is one that recognizes the impact of prior trauma exposure on health, on a patient's current medical/mental health status, and on coping style and engagement with clinical care.[3] TIC additionally recognizes that the medical system infrastructure, including patient-provider power differentials and medical interventions may be experienced as traumatic.[3] Finally, TIC implementation in the clinical setting, through staff TIC training, mentorship, and patient TIC education, has been associated with increased patient care satisfaction with improved engagement in disposition planning and increased staff workplace satisfaction.[17]

CONCEPTUALIZING TRAUMA-INFORMED CARE USING ETHICAL FRAMEWORKS

TIC is aligned with feminist, narrative, and principlist ethical theory and methodology, and understanding these approaches can assist clinicians and clinician-ethics consultants alike in understanding and implementing sound clinical care that respects patients' unique characteristics and personal values. These ethical lenses, in particular, both highlight the ethical importance of TIC itself as well as have the potential to assist in generating potential courses of intervention for patients in light of often competing personal and clinical considerations. Understanding the contributions of these approaches in identifying and seeking to end oppression, situating treatment and care in the context of an individual's lived experience and personal story, and creating both a willingness and commitment to balancing competing ethical priorities in the care of individuals and the design of systems, is central to the enterprise of person-centered care embodied in TIC.

First, feminist ethics aims "to understand, critique, and correct how gender operates within our moral beliefs, practices and our methodological approaches to ethical theory."[18] Feminist theories of intersectionality have broadened the scope of feminist ethics to consider the complex identities of individuals and groups, with varying potential impacts of race, gender, education, income, and culture/ethnicity in societal perceptions of power and privilege.[18] Feminist ethics has concerned itself with the existence of societal systems that create and perpetuate oppression, the constraints placed on specific persons due to their affiliation with particular societal groups.[19] Feminist ethics squarely informs TIC because trauma itself is more prevalent in and commonly experienced by individuals from marginalized societal groups, and may further marginalize and oppress those affected through intensification of powerlessness and a loss of agency.[20] Given the prevalence of trauma in marginalized populations, including persons with mental illness, an ethical lens sensitive to oppression is critical for a trauma-informed ethics and approach to care. Simply stated, feminist ethics recognizes the moral priority of establishing voice and empowerment for persons who are silenced and marginalized.

Feminist ethics additionally considers the network of complex social relationships within which moral norms develop and moral dilemmas arise.[19] Prioritizing the relational nature of ethics has led to the development of care ethics, in which moral agents are perceived as responding to the care needs of self and others with compassion and empathy.[21] Within the medical context, care ethics can facilitate relationally influenced moral determinations, with inclusion and integration of both patient and provider perspectives, promoting patient safety, agency, and therapeutic alliance.[21] Care ethics situates decisions about clinical treatment in the context of subjective and objective dimensions of care rather than striving to justify treatment interventions based on abstract or academic norms. Specifically, care ethics aligns with TIC by placing the question of what it would mean and what it would look like for a person to be "cared for," "cared about," and "taken care of" in the context of their individual lived experience, personal history, and ways of making meaning for their life.[21] TIC explicitly uses a relational focus, as exposure to trauma can adversely impact interpersonal relationships, with disempowerment and disconnection from social supports.[3] TIC and the ethics of care framework both foster rebuilding relationships, with TIC highlighting peer support and creation of collaborative partnerships.[3,19]

Formation of trusting relationships with care providers achieved through TIC may also facilitate the therapeutic use of patient narratives in TIC. In contrast to a trauma-specific framework, where reconstruction and integration of the trauma narrative are components of trauma therapy, the use of narrative in TIC may be an important tool in understanding patient history and experience toward an effective and therapeutic treatment plan for the whole person, not just the identified medical condition of concern in the clinical encounter.[20] In this respect, TIC draws from the foundations of narrative ethics, which aims to understand patient and family narratives to appreciate how they relate to moral dilemmas and distress.[22] Narrative ethics both assists and supports patients and/or families in sharing personal history, lived experience, and accounts of developing an understanding of their values, preferences, and coping strategies to identify morally permissible choices to manage moral dilemmas/distress.[22] Narrative ethics is aligned with TIC, as it may empower trauma survivors to discuss their experiences of care and share stories that are empowering to them as they may relate to their care values and goals.[22] Narrative approaches can foster empathic understanding and collaborative care alliance to arrive at patient-centered moral judgments and care outcomes.[22] By doing so, narrative ethics both informs the approach of TIC to the patient and supports the importance of TIC itself in centering care on the patient and the patient's experience.

TIC may also be situated in the principlist theory of Beauchamp and Childress,[23] which in its focus on balancing among 4 key moral principles to guide ethical decision making, has perhaps become the dominant paradigm in western biomedical ethics over the past 40 years. The principlism of Beauchamp and Childress[23] identifies 4 equal moral principles: (1) Autonomy: the right to self-governance achieved through respect for autonomous decision making; (2) Beneficence: the promotion of the welfare of others; (3) Nonmaleficence: the duty not to harm; and (4) Justice: fair allocation of scarce medical resources, such as access to high-quality medical care.[23] Through identification of how these principles manifest in the facts and circumstances of individual cases, principlism allows for a balancing of considerations in developing morally permissible courses of treatment from among which individual preferences and values may be used to determine clinical interventions. This ethical approach may serve to undergird the TIC commitments to recognizing and empowering individuals' decisions (autonomy), avoiding harm (nonmaleficence) and providing competent care (beneficence), and addressing how the design of systems may allocate care to individuals affected by trauma (justice). Specifically, TIC approaches highlight the need to foster safe, transparent, and collaborative care environments to promote patient agency in their clinical decision making.[3] TIC is, therefore, centered on the promotion of autonomy, as providing capable decision makers with medical information to make choices in accordance with their personal values and preferences, promotes transparency, and places the locus of control with the patient during an episode of care.[3] Health care systems promoting autonomy are also beneficent, as the opportunity to choose one's preferred care option, aligned with personal values, promotes a sense of safety and well-being. TIC practices aim to provide care that minimizes retraumatization and distress associated with care interventions, demonstrating nonmaleficence.[10] This aim may be achieved through open communication between patients and care providers, involvement of peer/family supports, offering choices and opportunities for taking control wherever feasible, practices promoting beneficence, and reducing harm.[10] Finally, TIC aims to minimize health disparities by offering care services responsive to the needs of members of historically marginalized and oppressed groups, who commonly experience trauma.[3] By fostering a health infrastructure that provides accessible, responsive care to diverse patient populations, TIC embodies the principle of just allocation of care resources.

Clinical Vignette

During your evaluation of Ms E, she reports a history of childhood sexual abuse, with a history of complex PTSD. She identifies the anniversary of her perpetrator's death as a pre-admission trigger, with intensified nightmares, flashbacks, and distress. She links her worsened PTSD symptoms to the foreign body insertion, which she identifies as a coping strategy to manage her distress. She describes her fear of medical settings and her history of being placed in physical restraints during a prior hospitalization. Ms E disagrees with her mother's decision to bring her to the hospital. Despite repeated explanations and attempts to support Ms E in understanding the potentially significant health risks of refusing treatment, Ms E continues to deny these risks, including infection, sepsis, and death. She bases her own assessment on prior personal experience of foreign body insertion, which did not result in any medical harm.

You acknowledge Ms E's unease and anxiety about being in the hospital, and at the same time note your concern with her fever, rising white cell count, and the medical need for further care. You explore the importance of her relationship with her mother, who is concerned for her well-being. You discuss that although Ms E has an understanding of her recent medical events, there is significant discrepancy between her appraisal of her current medical risks and that of her treating physician. You propose a shared decision-making model with both the patient and her mother involved in decision making. Ms E is amenable to involve her mother in her care and notes that she would receive this arrangement as a supportive one.

CONSENT AND CAPACITY CONSIDERATIONS IN TRAUMA-INFORMED CARE

Informed consent is an important component of clinical care, including TIC. Informed consent is the process by which a patient gives permission to a physician or other clinical team member to do something to or for them so as to provide medical care. Informed consent places the patient in the position of authority about what happens to their body, provided that the patient has the ability to engage in the informed consent process. As such, informed consent empowers patients with knowledge regarding their clinical care, includes them as collaborators in the medical decision-making process, and minimizes provider-patient power differentials, promoting therapeutic alliance, trust, and transparency.[24] In the health care setting, patients must demonstrate the ability to provide informed consent, which includes demonstration of decisional capacity (with the presumption of capacity for adults) and the ability to make a voluntary decision.[24] Decisional capacity requires that 4 criteria are met: the ability to select a preferred treatment, to understand relevant medical information, to appreciate how this medical information relates to a specific medical condition and its treatment for the patient, and to provide a rationale for the preferred medical treatment.[25] Patients with past history of trauma and/or psychiatric disorders are presumed capable of making treatment decisions, yet the specific clinical, affective, and behavioral circumstances of a clinical encounter may draw capacity into question either related to a specific treatment intervention or all aspects of care including treatment itself. In these circumstances, a capacity assessment is required to determine the patient's ability to make decisions about proposed medical treatments.

Patients with decisional capacity and the ability to provide informed consent may refuse routine and emergency medical treatment in accordance with their autonomous goals and values.[26] Patients who lack decisional capacity, and therefore cannot provide informed consent, however, require the assistance of a surrogate decision maker, with medical decisions ideally based on known prior capacitated wishes of the patient.[27] For patients deemed incapacitated to make a specific treatment decision, especially patients with a history of trauma, the loss of the ability and right to choose a preferred care intervention may precipitate disempowerment and retraumatization, contrary to the core principles and commitments of TIC. Removal of decision-making ability may then perpetuate the experience of trauma and distrust of medical providers, potentially contributing to care nonadherence and disengagement.[13] A trauma-informed lens, therefore, presents an imperative to minimize disempowerment if not empower trauma survivors who have been found to be decisionally incapacitated with respect to a particular medical intervention.[3]

One approach to promote empowerment for decisionally incapacitated patients is shared decision making. Shared decision making refers to collaborative communication between patients and providers, where information relevant to a specific medical decision is exchanged and patients are supported in making informed care choices.[28] The shared decision-making model rests on provider provision of medical information and relevant treatment options or "choice talk," detailed review of the risks/benefits of potential treatment options or "option talk," and supporting patients in their consideration of this information, combined with their values and preferences, to formulate an informed medical decision or "decision talk."[28] A shared decision-making framework is of value in a trauma-informed context because rather than excluding the incapacitated patient from participation in decisions and potentially retraumatizing the patient, shared decision making promotes the patient's voice and empowerment, works from the position of supporting strengths rather than highlighting deficits, and keeps the patient central to the treatment decision making and interventions. In other words, increased understanding of potential positive and negative care consequences achieved though shared decision making may support patients in applying their personal preferences to medical treatment decisions, leading to empowered care choices.[28] Both capacitated and incapacitated patients may be included in a shared decision-making model. Incapacitated patients may be encouraged to share their care preferences and values as they are able, with the support of a surrogate decision maker to ensure alignment of patient values and prior capable wishes with the preferred treatment choice. This approach is in contrast, for example, to approaches to incapacity that focus on the identification of a suitable surrogate to make decisions on behalf of a patient without full consideration of how the patient could be included. In addition, capacity evaluations are often an initial step in identifying the clinical and ethical parameters of medical treatment when there is disagreement between a patient and the treating physicians. However, although capacity evaluations are commonly an initial step in addressing an ethical dilemma, a determination of a lack of capacity for medical decision making does not permit treatment to automatically occur over a patient's objection.[29] In Ms E's case, for example, her impairment in the capacity appreciation standard is not synonymous with ethical permissibility to proceed with involuntary foreign body removal barring a life-threatening emergency. Instead, it is the beginning of a clinical-ethical deliberation that involves Ms E, her mother, and the clinical team to consider potential morally permissible courses of action, informed by Ms E's history, care needs, and treatment preferences. The potential risks and benefits of these morally permissible actions must be weighed, with her history of trauma an important factor in this risk-benefit appraisal. Because trauma survivors may have experienced coercion, disempowerment, and betrayal of trust, medical procedures that precipitate reexperience of past trauma may be associated with significant distress and potential mental health destabilization.[13] Consequently, such significant risks must be carefully considered by the provider and patient in collaboration to arrive at clinically and morally permissible treatment decisions.

Clinical Vignette

The medical team, including you, holds a family meeting with Ms E and her mother to review the risks and benefits of various treatment options, including discharge home with no treatment, continued medical monitoring in the hospital, and/or foreign body removal by the gynecology service. Ms E states that she does not wish to prolong her hospital admission, and strongly prefers to be discharged. Her mother states that she wants Ms E to remain in the hospital for care, and that she is not comfortable having her return home without foreign body removal. Ms E expresses significant frustration with the experience of being controlled. Ms E is supported in the use of affect regulation strategies, including deep breathing and taking a break from the meeting. After about an hour, the group reconvenes. Ms E. indicates that she feels uncomfortable with her current care team in the hospital, does not want to be in the hospital, and is frightened that she will have to undergo forced foreign body removal, an intervention she identifies as highly traumatic. You review Ms E's goals of remaining healthy, set her goals as the treatment goals, and identify that foreign body removal is consistent with her stated preferences. Together you consider what might support her in undergoing an examination and foreign body removal to facilitate her stated goals of health and returning home. Ms E reports that having her mother present and having a female gynecologist would help. Ms E informs you that she will not undergo the procedure with a male physician.

A TRAUMA-INFORMED CARE APPROACH TO PATIENT REQUESTS FOR GENDER-SPECIFIC CLINICAL CARE

Requests for care providers of a preferred gender are complex and may be informed by a history of trauma exposure, religious and/or cultural preferences, and past clinical care experiences.[30] In particular, gender-concordant care may lead to reduced discomfort and unease during completion of history and physical examinations required for sexual, reproductive, and genitourinary health.[31] Care consistent with patient gender preferences may reduce the potential for retraumatization, and power differentials between patients and staff, especially for patients like Ms E who make specific requests in light of past traumatic events. However, these requests must be evaluated in the broad context of the institutional and societal setting for multiple reasons, including both practical and ethical considerations.[32]

When confronted with gender-specific care requests, clinicians are required to weigh competing moral obligations.[31] Respecting autonomous preferences to refuse care from clinicians of specific genders may promote patient empowerment, sense of safety ,and be consistent with beneficent care based on patient values and goals.[31] Key care considerations for nonmaleficence include the urgency of the recommended clinical treatment, with an important potential reason for request refusal, requirement for emergency medical care, without which patient health outcomes would be compromised.[31] Justice and fairness-related moral concerns include obligations to provide just care to patients from marginalized groups or identities, the medical needs of the community served, and the medical community, with equitable employment and education for male/female/nonbinary identified medical trainees and providers.[31] In addition, in considering gender-specific care requests of patients, the potential discriminatory effects on staff and in the workplace should also be considered.[32]

A trauma-informed lens may assist with appraisal of core ethical obligations. From a TIC perspective, collaborative communication is critical, and care team members may facilitate understanding and communication by exploring a patient's reasons for gender-specific care requests, addressing care concerns and perceived power-imbalances, and considering accommodations to support medical treatment.[31] Safety is a core feature of TIC and requests for gender-specific care linked to nonmaleficence and reducing potential harms through retraumatization and significant psychological distress are important, especially for patients with marginalized social identities associated with reduced decision-making power in their lives; prioritizing patient autonomous requests with choice and control in their care may have substantial benefits for beneficence and trust in medical care provision, as well as justice.[10,31] Emergency care requirements or community centers with reduced numbers of providers, may not be able to meet gender-specific care requests. Transparency is critical to promote trust, with empathic disclosure and consideration of harm-reduction strategies; having a friend/family member present, a preferred gender clinician in the room, or hospital transfer/care referral.[10,31]

Clinical Vignette

The care team meets to review Ms E's care. Given the absence of an acute life-threatening medical concern and the risk of severe trauma from involuntary treatment, involuntary removal of the foreign body is determined to be neither clinically nor ethically appropriate. The gynecology consultant, however, makes the clinical recommendation that although foreign body removal is indicated, it is not emergent. Therefore, although removal at that time is recommended, there could also be the option of removal at a future time with familiar female clinical staff members should Ms E refuse and should her clinical condition remain stable. On reassessment several hours later, Ms E informs you that she has decided to undergo the examination with a female provider and her mother present. Following the examination and foreign body removal, Ms E expresses relief. She reports experiencing mild distress during the examination and that it had gone better than expected. She notes distress about her use of foreign body insertion as a coping strategy, with commitment to ongoing work with her outpatient mental health team. She relays appreciation for the understanding, patience, and care from her clinical team at the hospital and gratitude for being empowered to participate in her care choices rather than receiving coercive or involuntary care and restraint as she had in the past. Ms E highlights the impact of this past treatment experience as negatively affecting her ability to receive medical treatment and engage with medical teams. You support her use of coping strategies and collaborative work during this admission.

INVOLUNTARY TREATMENT CONSIDERATIONS IN TRAUMA-INFORMED CARE

Involuntary treatment is common in clinical practice and may take a variety of forms, including involuntary hospitalization and/or medication administration, use of open and/or locked-door seclusion, and physical and/or chemical restraints, among the most common forms of involuntary interventions in acute medical and psychiatric settings.[26] Restraint use has been associated with physical harms, such as compromised cardiorespiratory functioning and potential for asphyxia.[33] Psychological harms of involuntary treatment include negative relationships with staff in the setting of experience of medical practices as coercive and punitive, and negative views of self, such as loss of control, dignity, and self-respect during care.[34]

TIC principles highlight that a safe physical and psychological environment is critical to promoting the well-being and recovery of trauma survivors.[3] TIC models highlight that forcible, involuntary treatment has the potential to pose harms to trauma survivors through precipitation of the reexperience of past trauma and emotional distress through disempowerment and coercion.[35] Betrayal trauma, related to the experience of trust violation in an interpersonal relationship, has been linked to reduced trust in physicians and health care systems, and nonadherence to medical care recommendations.[13] Given the existing link between trauma exposure, mistrust and care nonadherence, use of coercive practices may pose harms through producing new traumatic experiences, worsening mistrust of medical systems, and further avoidance and care nonadherence behaviors.[13] The use of involuntary treatment is also potentially traumatic for staff members who witness or are involved in these practices and may experience vicarious trauma.[10]

State, federal, and international-level organizations, such as the National Association of State Mental Health Program Directors (NASMHPD), have championed initiatives to minimize involuntary treatment.[36] Seclusion and restraint prevention tools including staff training in deescalation and TIC approaches, identification of individuals at high risk of violence, and development of individualized patient behavioral treatment plans have been implemented to reduce involuntary care.[36] Debriefing immediately following acute episodes of restraint/seclusion with a subsequent care review with the treatment team can promote knowledge development to inform continued policies and procedures to reduce these events over time.[36] Debriefing is also intended to support staff and reduce the potential traumatic impact of such events on involved medical personnel.[36] Organizational leadership, health consumer advocacy for restraint/seclusion reduction, and continuous data collection and monitoring are additional prevention strategies.[36] For example, implementation of these NASMHPD strategies on inpatient psychiatry units has been shown to reduce patient time in restraints and seclusion, with implementation fidelity variable over time, highlighting the need to monitor successful implementation.[37] Reduction in restraint and seclusion use has also been associated with reduced health care costs with reduction in staff sick time, staff turnover, and reduced patient and staff injuries.[38]

Clinical Vignette

While you finish your documentation, Ms E's nurse pulls you aside. She tells you that she was part of a behavioral code during her prior shift and assisted in restraining a patient and administering intramuscular (IM) medication. She reports being preoccupied and distressed about her involvement in restraining this patient. She expresses that the patient's treatment was contrary to her being a caring and compassionate provider. She discloses her own history of physical trauma and that this clinical event was retraumatizing for her. She has requested the remainder of the day off for an urgent appointment with her own mental health specialist and to prioritize self-care amidst her current level of distress. She requests your assistance to arrange a debrief to review the event, which you agree to facilitate with the unit charge nurse.

TRAUMA-INFORMED CARE AND PREVENTIVE ETHICS: VICARIOUS TRAUMATIZATION AND TRAUMA-INFORMED CARE BARRIERS AND IMPLEMENTATION

TIC recognizes the impact of trauma on both patients and their care providers, actively promoting the safety and well-being of both patients and staff.[3] Vicarious traumatization refers to "negative changes in the clinicians' view of self, others, and the world resulting from repeated empathic engagement with patients' trauma-related thoughts, memories, and emotions."[39] Vicarious trauma is the consequence of chronic, indirect exposure to distressing trauma narratives, with increased risk associated with individual factors, including providers with a personal history of trauma and mental health concerns; patient care factors, such as high trauma patient caseloads; and occupational factors, including limited access to peer supervision and support.[40] Vicarious trauma may also occur in patients witnessing traumatic events while receiving care.[39] Secondary trauma exposure in the workplace is considered an occupational psychological hazard, which may progress to PTSD.[39] Vicarious trauma has also been associated with reduced provider wellness, burnout and high workplace employee turnover and reduced continuity and quality of patient care.[41] An absence of TIC, with use of practices such as restraints and seclusion, can contribute to both direct patient trauma and vicarious trauma for involved staff members, negatively shaping provider cognitions around safety, control, and trust in the workplace.[10]

TIC approaches are aligned with preventive ethics in their aim to recognize the widespread exposure to trauma within patient and provider populations and to implement universal workplace strategies to mitigate the harms of new patient/provider traumas, retraumatization events, and secondary trauma exposure.[3] Although TIC has been associated with increased patient care engagement and increased staff well-being, there are barriers to its implementation.[10,17]

TIC implementation barriers may be broadly conceptualized as occurring at the health system, institutional, and individual provider levels.[10] At the health system level, shortages of mental health care providers, and absence of adequate mental health care funding, with competing public health initiatives, can reduce funding and staffing to support TIC implementation.[10] At the organizational level, absence of adequate staff supervision and training in TIC, a risk aversive culture implementing coercive and controlling practices, high staff turnover, and significant administrative task burden may overwhelm providers and reduce the time available for them to engage in clinical activities, training initiatives, and care supervision.[10] Individual-level barriers may include gaps in provider knowledge of the extent of trauma exposure and its impact on physical and mental health, reluctance to shift from biomedical to biopsychosocial models to incorporate social and psychological supports for patients and staff, and provider burnout and personal and/or workplace trauma exposures.[10]

Moving toward TIC implementation in health care settings requires a multilevel approach spanning legislative, institutional, and individual provider advocacy interventions.[3] Advocacy from organizational/state and community leaders aligned with trauma and recovery is needed to champion TIC initiatives and support allocation of funding to TIC resources.[3] Organizational TIC policies, available to patients and staff for review, are needed to promote safety in the workplace with commitment to collaborative care, reduced involuntary practices, and trauma screening.[3] Medical and mental health staff require training in TIC and conducting a basic trauma assessment, with basic skills to support patients and knowledge of how to collaborate with local mental health providers.[3] Screening tools for patient experience of trauma include the life events checklist for the DSM-5 and the trauma assessment for adults, with resources for vicarious trauma in providers, including the impact of event scale and secondary traumatic stress scale.[39,42] Prioritization of TIC implementation must be sustained over time with progress monitoring, quality assurance tracking, and evaluation measures in place within the organization to monitor adherence to TIC screening, training initiatives, and reduction of traumatic practices over time.[3]

SUMMARY

Embedding TIC practices within hospital policies and routine clinical care has the potential to mitigate the adverse effects of trauma on patient safety, care engagement, and provider wellness. TIC aims to promote patient agency and safety, and reduce retraumatization, are aligned with ethical principles promoting autonomy, benefi-cence, and nonmaleficence. Prioritizing care provision that meets the needs of histor-ically traumatized and marginalized groups promotes justice and is consistent with feminist ethical frameworks. The pervasive nature of trauma requires simultaneous use of interventions focusing on acknowledging the impact of trauma and minimizing its adverse effects, as well as those focused on curbing the growing incidence of trau-matic experiences on individual, community, and global scales. Given the interwoven relationships among marginalization, trauma, and health, efforts to reduce the impact and incidence of trauma will inevitably promote physical and mental well-being.

CLINICS CARE POINTS

- All mental health and medical care providers can participate in advocating for and creating a trauma informed care environment that can be universally implemented across patient care settings.

- Routine trauma exposure screening should be considered to optimize trauma informed care practices across medical and mental health care settings.

- Policies aligned with trauma informed care principles, such as those aimed to minimize restraint and seclusion use, require provider advocacy and continued vigilance to policy adherence over time.

- Care provider wellness initiatives, including screening for vicarious trauma and accessible provider mental health supports, are central to the creation of a trauma-informed clinical care setting.

DISCLOSURE

The author has nothing to disclose.

REFERENCES

1. Benjet C, Bromet E, Kessler RC, et al. The epidemiology of traumatic event expo-sure worldwide: results from the World Mental Health Survey Consortium. Psychol Med 2016;46(2):327–43.
2. Kimberg L, Wheeler M. Chapter 2: trauma and trauma informed care. In: Gerber MR, editor. Trauma informed health care approaches. . Cham, Switzerland: Springer Nature Switzerland AG; 2019. p. 25–56.
3. The Substance Abuse and Mental Health Services Administration (SAMHSA). SAMHSA's Concept of trauma and guidance for a trauma-informed approach. SAMHSA's trauma and justice strategic initiative. 2014. Available at: https://ncsacw.samhsa.gov/userfiles/files/SAMHSA_Trauma.pdf. Accessed April 21, 2021.
4. American Psychiatric Association. The diagnostic and statistical manual. 5th edi-tion. Washington, DC: American Psychiatric Publishing; 2013.
5. Gerber MR, Gerber EB. Chapter 1: an introduction to trauma and health. In: Gerber MR, editor. Trauma informed health care approaches. Cham, Switzerland: Springer Nature Switzerland AG; 2019.
6. Ford E, Bergmann MM, Boeing H, et al. Healthy lifestyle behaviors and all-cause mortality among adults in the United States. Prev Med 2012;55(1):23–7.
7. Felitti V, Nordenberg D, Williamson DF, et al. Relationship of childhood abuse and household dysfunction to many of the leading causes of death in adults. Am J Prev Med 1998;14(4):245–58.

8. Huckshorn K, Lebel J. Chapter 5: trauma informed care. In: Yeager K, Cutler D, Svendsen D, et al, editors. Modern community mental health: an interdisciplinary approach. New York, NY: Oxford University Press; 2013. p. 62–83.

9. Subica AM, Claypoole KH, Wylie AM, et al. PTSD's mediation of the relationship between trauma, depression, substance use, mental health and physical health in individuals with severe mental illness: evaluating a comprehensive model. Schizophr Res 2012;136:104–9.

10. Sweeney A, Filson B, Kennedy A, et al. A paradigm shift: relationships in trauma-informed mental health services. BJPsych Adv 2018;24:319–33.

11. Cusack KJ, Grubaugh AL, Knapp RG, et al. Unrecognized trauma and PTSD among public mental health consumers with chronic and severe mental illness. Community Ment Health J 2006;42(5):487–500.

12. Watson P. PTSD as a public mental health priority. Curr Psychiatry Rep 2019; 21:61.

13. Klest B, Tamaian A, Boughner E, et al. A model exploring the relationship between betrayal trauma and health: the roles of mental health, attachment, trust in healthcare systems, and non-adherence to treatment. Psychol Trauma 2019; 11(6):656–62.

14. Roberts AL, Gilman SW, Breslau J, et al. Race/ethnic differences in exposure to traumatic events, development of post-traumatic stress disorder, and treatment seeking for post-traumatic stress disorder in the United States. Psychol Med 2011;41(1):71–83.

15. Hopper E, Bassuk EL, Oliver J, et al. Shelter from the storm: trauma-informed care in homeless services settings. Open Health Serv Policy J 2010;3:80–100.

16. Klest B. Childhood trauma, poverty and adult victimization. Psychol Trauma 2012; 4(93):245–51.

17. Hales TW. Trauma informed care outcome study. Res Soc Work Pract 2019;29(5): 529–39.

18. Norlock K. Feminist ethics: the Stanford encyclopedia of philosophy. 2019. Available at: https://plato.stanford.edu/entries/feminism-ethics/. Accessed April 12, 2021.

19. Sherwin S. No longer patient. Feminist, ethics and health care. Philadelphia, PA: Temple University Press; 1992.

20. Herman J. Trauma and recovery. New York, NY: Basic Books, a Member of the Perseus Book Group; 1992.

21. Timmons M. Moral theory: an introduction. 2nd Ed. Lanham, MD: Rowman & Littlefield; 2013.

22. Montello M. Narrative ethics. Narrative ethics: the role of stories in bioethics, special report. Hastings Cent Rep 2014;44(1):S2–6.

23. Beauchamp TL, Childress JF. Principles of biomedical ethics. 7th edition. New York, NY: Oxford University Press; 2013.

24. Sher Y, Sermsak L. Ethical issues: capacity to make medical decisions. Psychiatric times. 2014. Available at: http://www.psychiatrictimes.com/special-reports/ethical-issues-patients-capacity-make-medical-decisions/page/0/1. Accessed March 9 2021.

25. Appelbaum P. Assessment of patients' competence to consent to treatment. N Engl J Med 2007;357:1834–40.

26. Glezer A, Brendel RW. Beyond emergencies: the use of physical restraints in medical and psychiatric settings. Harv Rev Psychiatry 2010;18(6):353–8.

27. Torke A, Alexander GC, Lantos J, et al. Substituted judgement: the limitations of autonomy in surrogate decision making. J Gen Intern Med 2008;23(9):1514–7.

28. Elwyn G. Shared decision making: a model for clinical practice. J Gen Intern Med 2012;27(10):1361–7.
29. Kontos N. Beyond capacity: identifying ethical dilemmas underlying capacity evaluation requests. Psychosomatics 2013;54:103–10.
30. Waseem M, Miller A. Requests for a male or female physician. AMA J Ethics 2008;10(7):429–33.
31. Peek M, Lo B, Fernandez A, et al. How should physicians respond when patient's distrust them because of their gender? AMA J Ethics 2017;19(4):332–9.
32. American Medical Association. Report of the Council on Ethical and Judicial Affairs. 2020. Available at: https://www.ama-assn.org/system/files/2020-12/nov2020-ceja-report-1.pdf. Accessed May 18, 2021.
33. Barnett R, Stirling C, Pandyan AD, et al. A review of the scientific literature related to the adverse impact of physical restraint. Med Sci Law 2012;52:137–42.
34. Hughes R, Hayward M, Finlay WML, et al. Patient's perceptions of the impact of involuntary patient care on self, relationships and recovery. J Ment Health 2009; 18(2):152–60.
35. Watson S, Thorburn K, Everett M, et al. Care without coercion—mental health rights, personal recovery and trauma informed care. Aust J Soc Issues 2014; 49(4):529–53.
36. National Associated of State Mental Health Program Directors (NASMHPD). Six core strategies for reducing seclusion and restraint use. 2006. Available at: https://www.nasmhpd.org/sites/default/files/Consolidated%20Six%20Core%20Strategies%20Document.pdf. Accessed March 1, 2021.
37. Wieman D, Camacho-Gonsalves T, Huckshorn KA, et al. Multisite study of an evidence-based practice to reduce seclusion and restrain in psychiatric inpatient facilities. Psychiatr Serv 2014;65(3):345–51.
38. Lebel J, Goldstein R. The economic cost of using restraint and the value added by restraint reduction or elimination. Psychiatr Serv 2005;56:1109–14.
39. Quitangon G. Vicarious trauma in clinicians: fostering resilience and preventing burnout. Psychiatric Times 2019;36(7):18–9.
40. Newell J, MacNeil G. Professional burnout, vicarious trauma, secondary traumatic stress and compassion fatigue: a review of theoretical terms, risk factors, and preventative methods for clinicians and researchers. Best Pract Ment Health Int J 2010;6(2):57–68.
41. Boscarino JA, Adams RE, Figley CR, et al. Secondary trauma issues for psychiatrists. Psychiatr Times 2010;27(11):24–6.
42. US Department of Veterans Affairs. National Center for PTSD. Trauma exposure measures. Available at: https://www.ptsd.va.gov/professional/assessment/te-measures/index.asp. Accessed May 4, 2021.

Autonomy and Multiculturalism

Kaila Rudolph, MD, MPH, MBE[a,b,c,]*

KEYWORDS

• Autonomy • Culture • Psychiatry • Clinical ethics

KEY POINTS

- Patient and provider cultural affiliations can have a significant impact on their preferred mental health decision-making models, definitions and explanations of psychiatric symptoms, and preferred treatment modalities.
- The traditional Western individualist conception of respect for autonomy may produce patient and family distress for those affiliated with more collectivist cultures whereby relational autonomy and close familial involvement are central to navigating clinical care choices.
- Use of standardized cultural assessment tools, such as the *Diagnostic and Statistical Manual of Mental Disorders* (Fifth Edition) cultural formulation interview, may assist providers in preemptively addressing cultural challenges in the mental health care setting and ensuring decision-making preferences are discussed with patient and families in advance of treatment decision making.
- Given the growing cultural diversity within the US population, continued advocacy for integration of multicultural practices within psychiatric care settings, such as formation of provider-community cultural partnerships, is needed.

AUTONOMY AND MULTICULTURALISM: ETHICAL CONSIDERATIONS IN PSYCHIATRIC PRACTICE
Defining Autonomy

The ethical principle, respect for autonomy, has become a cornerstone of Western medical ethics. The American Psychiatric Association identifies honoring patient autonomous preferences, through practices such as informed consent, as an imperative in the ethical practice of medicine.[1] The principlism framework of Beauchamp and Childress,[2] recognizes respect for autonomy as 1 of 4 prima facie principles of medical ethics, highlighting moral obligations to provide individual patients with the opportunity for self-governance, to formulate medical decisions and select preferred

[a] Department of Consultation-Liaison, Boston Medical Center, Boston, MA, USA; [b] Department of Geriatric Psychiatry, Boston Medical Center, Boston, MA, USA; [c] Department of Psychiatry, Boston University School of Medicine, Boston, MA, USA
* Doctor's Office Building, 720 Harrison Avenue, Suite 7600, Boston, MA 02118, USA.
E-mail address: Kaila.Rudolph@bmc.org

Psychiatr Clin N Am 44 (2021) 537–548
https://doi.org/10.1016/j.psc.2021.08.006
0193-953X/21/© 2021 Elsevier Inc. All rights reserved.

medical treatments in accordance with their personal values and preferences. Autonomous decision making requires that an individual act in a manner that demonstrates decision making with the following: (1) Intentional, deliberate, and consistent with a formulated action plan; (2) understanding adequate knowledge of information required to make the proposed choice; and (3) noncontrol, decisions made in the absence of undue pressure or coercive influence.[2] As respect for autonomy has grown in prominence, particularly in the Western medical setting, there has been increased focus on shared decision making, characterized by collaborative information exchange between physicians and patients to support patient-informed care choices.[3] The goal of shared decision-making models is to blend evidence-based medical expertise, information the physician conveys through informed consent to provide information a reasonable patient would deem necessary, with individual patient's expertise regarding their own values, preferences, and health care goals.[3] Provision of medical information serves to enhance patient understanding and increase autonomous medical decision-making capacity.[4]

Recognition of the influence of relationships, such as the patient-physician dyad, on understanding and capacity to exercise one's autonomous capability, has led to a transition from focusing on the individual as an independent decision maker, to models prioritizing relational influences on autonomy.[2] Relational autonomy recognizes that individual decision makers exist within complex social networks, with family and community affiliations, and social factors, such as ethnicity, culture, and gender, shaping one's identity, core values, and preferences, features increasingly recognized as being central to the development of decision-maker choices.[4] Rather than being seen as independent, in relational models, decision makers are conceptualized as persons embedded within a broad interpersonal context with interdependence upon others to share responsibilities, such as medical care provision, and shape how decisions are conceptualized and which treatment is ultimately selected.[4] Medical providers must balance the duality that exists between conceptualizing patients as free from significant social influence upon decision making to patients operating in complex interdependent relationships that have a high degree of involvement and influence on and importance to patient choice.[4]

Defining Autonomy Within a Cultural Context

Concepts of personhood and autonomy have been shown to vary across ethnicity and culture.[2,5] For example, a study of ethnically diverse adults in the United States aged 65 and older regarding attitudes on diagnosis and disclosure of terminal illness found that Korean and Mexican Americans were significantly more likely to prefer nondisclosure of the diagnosis to the patient and to favor family involvement in medical decision making, as compared with European and African Americans.[2,5] This finding highlights the broad spectrum of patient decision-making preferences, and the importance of health care provider elicitation of these attitudes, values, and preferences. In general, patients may align most with 1 of 3 general approaches to medical decision making: (1) Collectivist, family-oriented models, prioritizing the impact of one's illness and medical course on family with a high-degree of family involvement; (2) a combination of family and individual considerations requiring promotion of patient autonomy in balance with traditional family values; and (3) individualist models focused primarily on individual patient care needs.[5,6] These preferences may change over time, requiring provider reassessment, in the context of factors such as emergent illness and functional dependence, and for persons who have immigrated, the degree of acculturation to the new society.[6]

As the United States has become increasingly multicultural, with culturally, racially, and ethnically diverse groups and growing awareness of health care disparities across these domains, the importance of cultural considerations in health care has become a central focus in medicine.[7] The *Diagnostic and Statistical Manual of Mental Disorders* (Fifth Edition) (*DSM-5*) highlights incorporation of a patient's cultural context as essential for mental health assessment, diagnosis, and treatment.[8] Culture is defined as the "systems of knowledge, concepts, rules, practices that are learned and transmitted across generations."[8] Culture may incorporate domains, such as language, religion, family traditions, and structure, and is dynamic, with cultural norms and practices evolving over time.[8] Exposure to multiple cultural influences is common, and it is important to approach each person as holding unique personal beliefs and identity, with avoidance of overgeneralizations pertaining to groups that may share similar characteristics, such as those of the same race or gender, given the highly heterogeneous nature of culture even within groups sharing common traits.[8] Accordingly, care providers, even if they share similar attributes with their patients, such as a common race and language, must remain attuned to cultural nuances that may affect mental health treatment.[8] The *DSM-5* has developed a short semistructured cultural formulation interview, to promote the systematic evaluation of cultural domains significant for mental health care. It focuses on the following: (1) The cultural definition of the presenting symptoms; (2) the cultural perceptions of the cause of the health concern and associated stressors and supports; (3) cultural factors influencing coping strategies and past help-seeking behavior; and (4) cultural factors impacting current help seeking behavior.[8] Standardized communication guides may minimize the potential influence of provider-implicit biases in cross-cultural care and preemptively address potential barriers to care engagement, including diverse values and care preferences, linguistic barriers, and cultural differences in illness explanatory models between patient and provider.[9]

Cultural evaluation and formulation are important components of the psychiatric assessment, as culture is associated with variations in mental health symptoms, understanding of illness cause, engagement in care, and preferred treatment modality.[10] Persons identifying with cultural minority groups may experience disproportionate exposure to social stressors, such as racism, discrimination, and for those who have immigrated, potential acculturation-related distress, which may affect mental health.[10] There is limited evidence that significant disparities in mental health diagnosis exist; however, higher rates of psychological symptoms have been found in minority populations, including higher rates of schizophrenia among African Americans, with the potential for cross-cultural diagnostic barriers affecting diagnostic accuracy.[11] Manifestations of stress and mental health symptoms are further influenced by cultural norms.[9] Communication practices and language to articulate emotional experience vary across cultures, with heterogenous conceptions of the relationship between mind and body and the potential for unique somatic symptoms to represent psychic distress across cultures.[10,11] Significant mental health care disparities have been noted across minority patient populations with respect to psychiatric care access and engagement in the United States.[11] For example, compared with whites, racial and ethnic minorities are less likely to access mental health services, are more likely to receive poorer quality care, and have higher rates of premature treatment termination.[11] Mental health stigma, insurance and financial barriers, limited access to traditional remedies within Western contexts, and provider discrimination may be potential contributors to the existing mental health care disparities.[11]

Cultural competence, cultural humility, and patient-centered care have emerged as medical concepts highlighting the need to respect the diversity of patient values and care preferences and to promote a respectful, inclusive, evidence-based care environment.[9] Cultural humility emphasizes the importance of a commitment to continual learning and self-improvement to develop one's capacity for honoring diverse cultural customs and values, whereas cultural competence emphasizes the development of skills to effectively understand one's own and others cultural perspectives and address this diversity effectively within patient and health care systems.[9] The term, "cultural competemility," has emerged from efforts to integrate competence and humility, considering both the process of humility and the outcome of competence together.[9] Cultural competemility requires clinicians "to maintain both an attitude and a lens of cultural competence and cultural humility as they engage in cultural encounters, obtain cultural knowledge, demonstrate the cultural skill of conducting a culturally sensitive cultural assessment, and become culturally aware of both their own biases and the presence of 'isms' (eg, racism, sexism)."[9] The emphasis on practitioner incorporation of cultural diversity into care practices is consistent with beneficent, nonmaleficent care, aligned with patient-stated values and preferences, that is attuned to justice, promoting access to high-quality care for minority populations. Cultural humility and competence in clinical care are critical considerations to address moral dilemmas that may arise when clinician and care provider systems are founded on cultural beliefs and values that vary from those of the patient.

Mirroring medical models increasingly focused on respect for cultural diversity, bioethics emphasizes the importance of culture on ethical norms influencing patient care preferences.[12] In contrast to moral universalism, which views moral principles as universal and independent of factors, such as cultural context, medical practitioners are encouraged to consider the manner and extent to which culture influences a particular patient's care.[7,13] Moral relativism posits that ethical standards should be considered relative to cultural context, with no absolute moral conventions or truths, such that each cultural group has equally valid frameworks for determining moral norms and how members within that group should behave.[13] This can translate to behaviors considered morally acceptable in 1 culture, deemed morally unacceptable in a different cultural context.[12] Restricted moral relativism continues to value cultural context, however, assumes that moral norms are subject to some universal constraints that are independent of culture, such as the general notion of not killing others, while continuing to allow for moral practices that may be specific to cultural context.[12] Ethical approaches recognizing some degree of moral diversity and multiculturalism are consistent with medicine's increased focus on integration of diverse cultural practices in the clinical setting. Cultural norms and values play a significant role in shaping patient medical decision-making models and treatment preferences.[14] Rigid adoption of Western norms, such as individualistic views of autonomy, may pose harms to patients through care that produces distress and tension within familial relationships and is fundamentally incompatible with patient values and beliefs, factors that may contribute to reduced care engagement and nonadherence, which may jeopardize patient health and further existing health care access disparities.[14]

Clinical Vignette

As the on-call psychiatrist at your hospital, you receive a page to assess Mr L, a patient admitted to the general medical ward. His primary medical team informs you that Mr L is a 73-year-old Chinese man, who immigrated to the United States 2 years ago with his wife, to reside with their adult daughter. He has no past psychiatric history and has been admitted for management of an acute exacerbation of his congestive heart failure. His clinical team notes concern that a concurrent depressive disorder may be adversely impacting his care adherence, given limited appetite, flat affect, social withdrawal, and recurrent vague somatic concerns, with no clear cause despite extensive medical workup. The team has attempted to discuss their concern for depression, with recommendation for antidepressant treatment, which Mr L has declined. The team is concerned with impaired understanding of his condition, with Mr L noting his condition is due to "flow" and "spirits." They request consultation to evaluate for an underlying psychiatric disorder, and as appropriate, his capacity to refuse any proposed psychiatric treatment. You clarify that Mr L speaks Mandarin and book an in-person interpreter.

On assessment with Mr L, his wife and daughter are present in the room, and he notes a preference to have them remain present for the evaluation. He articulates his challenges with heart failure and increased shortness of breath and fatigue, limiting his ability to help his family with household tasks, and go on daily walks, which he had previously enjoyed. He also notes missing his siblings and extended family in China since immigration to the United States. He reports concern with abdominal and back discomfort and persistent fatigue in addition to reduced appetite, energy, concentration, experience of burdening his family, and hopelessness about feasibility of returning home from hospital. He states he does not feel happy anymore. When discussing the cause of his feeling of unhappiness, guilt, and hopelessness, he discusses the influence of spirits impairing the flow of energy between his mind and body.[15] He is able to recall and demonstrate understanding of the antidepressant treatments discussed with his team earlier during admission and state their basic risks and proposed benefits, which he understands as promoting flow in his body. He remains uncertain about antidepressant treatment because of concern with polypharmacy and uncertainty whether it will be of benefit given his cardiac concerns. He does not endorse paranoid ideation or perceptual disturbance and exhibits a linear and organized thought process and intact orientation, attention, and memory. Collateral history from his wife and daughter notes that he has appeared increasingly dysphoric since his health challenges and immigration to the United States. They deny evidence of psychosis or memory impairment. You review his statements about spirits, and his daughter and wife note he has chronically mentioned these concerns around his medical challenges, noting such beliefs were endorsed by his parents and were common among his siblings.

Cultural Considerations in Capacity Evaluations

The moral duty to respect patient autonomy is met within the clinical context by honoring the autonomous preferences of persons with decision-making capacity, while ensuring that patients who do not meet decisional capacity thresholds, with inability to formulate decisions in accordance with their prior capable values and preferences, receive assistance from a substituted decision maker.[2] Capacity consultation requests rest on the cultural assumption that the person receiving treatment is the primary decision maker, acting independently from family or other supports.[2] This contrasts a relational conception of autonomy, with potential for an appointed family member or several persons jointly taking responsibility for medical decision making.[16] As Beauchamp and Childress[2] note, the moral obligation to respect patient autonomy is fulfilled through recognizing that patients have the ability to make choices regarding their care, including the decision whether they wish to make medical decisions and who should be appointed to assist with decision making in accordance with their preferences. As a component of routine medical practice, preemptively discussing how much information patients wish to receive and whether they, or an appointed decision maker, should work with their clinical team to discuss and provide consent for medical treatments is advised and consistent with respecting patient autonomy.[2] Such practices can avoid patient/family harms and distress, by reducing the likelihood of unwarranted capacity evaluations in a relational decision-making context, and avoidance of discussing medical information, such as risks of procedures, if a patient has noted they would find this distressing and have elected for family to receive this information.[16]

In addition to reduced applicability of patient capacity evaluations when patient and family are sharing decision-making responsibility, culture may impact the understanding and appreciation decisional capacity criteria.[16] Decisional capacity requires that patients demonstrate the following: (1) The ability to select a preferred treatment; (2) understanding of relevant medical information; (3) appreciation of how this medical information relates to their specific medical condition and its treatment; and (4) a rationale for the preferred medical treatment.[17] In a Western care context, understanding and appreciation criteria typically rely on illness models congruent with science and biology, with limited incorporation of religious or spiritual understandings of disease.[15,16] Consequently, patients like Mr L, who may hold long-standing beliefs that illness may be cause by factors outside of the realm of science, such as spirits or blockage in energy flow, may be deemed incapable because of failure to demonstrate understanding and appreciation consistent with Western norms.[15,16] Providers in these contexts may even be concerned about potential for psychotic symptoms.[16] Patients from diverse cultural contexts, wishing to make their own medical decisions, are at risk of being inaccurately deemed incapable because of limited provider incorporation of cultural factors in capacity evaluation.[16] This would violate the duty to respect autonomy, with associated harms from care incompatible with patient preferences and patient disempowerment and discrimination.

Culturally informed capacity evaluations, therefore, consider provider and patient cultural norms, with additional history from the patient and collateral informants to evaluate the impact of culture on understanding, appreciation, and ability to rationally manipulate relevant medical information.[18] Important aspects on clinical history include the following: (1) Past psychiatric history; (2) evidence of specific psychiatric symptoms or behavioral concerns impairing several functional domains; (3) the duration and nature of the beliefs held by the patient and (4) how these beliefs align with the patient's familial and larger cultural community; and (5) educational and socioeconomic background.[18] Consultation with patient's family members, a member of their cultural or religious community, and/or use of hospital resources, including interpreter services, spiritual care, and long-standing trusted members of their care team, such as a primary care physician, and hospital staff of similar cultural and/or ethnic background, may be helpful to provide an increased understanding of the role of culture in the patient's illness understanding and care preferences.[18] Inclusion of these supports in the capacity evaluation may also enhance patient sense of safety and provider understanding of patient responses in real-time during the capacity evaluation. The process of providing informed consent, obtaining psychiatric history, and capacity evaluation may also be completed over several meetings in hospital to ensure the necessary information and patient supports are provided.[18]

Thoughtful evaluation of patient preferences may also lead to a greater understanding of patient-preferred treatments and identification of any potential barriers to capacity, such as modification of provider language choices to ensure intended meaning is conveyed in a culturally appropriate manner and combining medical and cultural illness explanatory models with interdisciplinary involvement of medical and spiritual care teams.[18] In the case of Mr L, his statements about spirituality and energy flow were consistent with his baseline mental status and long-standing illness explanatory models, per patient and family, in the absence of evidence of psychosis, cognitive impairment, with intact ability to discuss antidepressant risks and benefits and provide a rationale for why he does not wish to pursue antidepressant treatment at this time. His evaluation was consistent with meeting the decisional capacity threshold to consent to and decline antidepressant treatment.

Clinical Vignette

The following morning, you receive a page from Mr L's primary medical team. They note that when discussing antidepressant treatment with Mr L, he continued to decline; however, his wife and daughter intervened, asked multiple questions about antidepressant treatment, and then strongly encouraged Mr L to accept antidepressant treatment, which he finally agreed to do. The primary medical team conveyed concern with family exerting a coercive influence upon Mr L's decision making, given that he has been assessed to have capacity to accept or refuse antidepressant treatment. They ask you to further clarify Mr L's treatment preferences and the role of family in these decisions.

You return with a Mandarin-speaking interpreter and evaluate Mr L in the absence of his family. He reports feeling very well supported by his family. He wishes for himself, his wife, and daughter to be involved in his medical decision making. He often feels fatigued in hospital and finds it helpful for family to clarify his medical information and discuss their treatment preferences. His notes that his wife is his primary care provider and discusses the significant impact that his illness has had on her. He is concerned about taking too many medications and is uncertain how much an antidepressant will assist him, however, acknowledges that antidepressant treatment is very important to his wife and daughter. He is amenable to trial antidepressant treatment, as the wishes and well-being of his family are very important to him, and he feels there is limited risk to trialing antidepressant medication. He reports very trusting relationships with his family in the absence of verbal, physical abuse, or neglect. You update his family and the medical team regarding this discussion, and antidepressant therapy is commenced.

Respect for Patient Autonomy: The Role of Family Involvement

The requirement that autonomous decision makers be free from controlling influences exerted by external factors, including the influence of other persons on the patient, poses challenges when moving from an individualist to relational conception of autonomy.[2,14] Given concern that patients in hospital may be vulnerable and distressed, with reduced ability to exercise their autonomy in the setting of acute illness, safeguards have emerged to protect patient autonomy from coercive influences, particularly from medical provider paternalism.[14] In the Western context, medical practitioners may promote independent patient decision making, as the patient is seen as being the most impacted by care decisions as they are the direct recipient of treatment, such that their preferences are prioritized.[14]

Family members, unlike medical providers, may be intimately involved in the patient's life, through shared activities, care provision, and strong attachment and care for their loved one, leading to personal investment in the patient's health and well-being.[14] The intimate nature of family relationships and common impact of patient illness on the patient and their family confer family with a greater understanding of the patient's illness and likelihood of common care goals shared by patient and family.[14] Given the impact of patient health and their medical decisions on their family members, health care decisions may be conceptualized as events impacting the entire family and appropriately considered within the relational realm.[14]

Although patient preferences for the degree of family involvement in their medical decision making may vary, in contrast to focusing on patient protection from external influences on decision making, some patients may prefer familial assistance.[14] Family support may be a relief to patients who may feel physically and emotionally burdened with health care information and decision-making pressures and may enhance patient sense of identity through preserved relationships and collaboration with family, and patients concerned with burdening their family may feel a reduced sense of responsibility with family involvement in their care decisions.[14] For patients and families electing to approach decision making collaboratively, provider efforts to maintain the patient as the individual decision maker may contribute to care misaligning with patient preferences and minimizing the impact of patient illness on family member well-being.[14] Respecting patient autonomy includes honoring how patients wish their medical decisions to be made, including prioritizing the preferences of family over their own.[14,19]

When patient and family care preferences are in conflict, with a discrepancy between patient-stated wishes and actions, as in the case of Mr L, care providers may consider meeting individually with the patient to (1) Clarify the extent of their preferred family involvement; (2) review any treatment preferences the patient may have, and how they wish to prioritize their preferences and family preferences; (3) review care aspects the patient may wish to maintain confidential; and (4) discuss the care plan, in accordance with patient wishes, in a family meeting.[19] In the Western setting, avoiding assumptions that patient decision making should occur independently or that family influence is consistent with coercion, while maintaining vigilant to any evidence of abuse, manipulation, or threatening behavior, toward the patient is important for honoring duties to respect patient autonomy.[19]

Clinical Vignette

While in hospital, Mr L's cardiac functioning is continuing to improve, and he has become increasingly engaged with clinical care. He has been adherent to antidepressant treatment in the absence of adverse effect. On your daily rounds, Mr L's nurse approaches you. She is holding several pills in her hand. She informs you that Ms L was administering these tablets to Mr L and identified them as herbal products. She asks you whether these should be administered alongside Mr L's other medications or whether Ms L should be informed to stop administering these to her husband.

On interview with Mr and Ms L, with the aid of a Mandarin-speaking interpreter, Ms L reported that she has been consulting an herbalist, who has prescribed several plant-based remedies for Mr L to target his fatigue and anorexia and promote strength. He has been receiving the herbal tablets twice daily for the past week in hospital. Mr L notes that he finds the herbal treatment helpful and wishes to continue their use in hospital and in the community, denying any adverse effects. You obtain the herbalist contact information from Ms L, with Mr and Ms L providing consent for you to obtain clinical information regarding the herbs prescribed. You also obtain the tablet box and ingredient list from Ms L and provide this to the inpatient pharmacist. The pharmacist reviews the ingredient list and notes that evidence is limited regarding the safety and efficacy of the prescribed herbal remedies. Collateral history from Mr L's herbalist is notable for limited evidence base and absence of Food and Drug Administration (FDA) approval for the prescribed remedies, with general tolerability and efficacy, in the absence of known adverse drug interactions, noted in the herbalist's clinical experience.

Patient Autonomy: Complementary and Alternative Medicine Considerations

Complementary and alternative medicine (CAM), which may include natural products and mind/body practices, is commonly used within the United States, with estimates that roughly one-third of households in the United States have used complementary medical treatments.[20] CAM may represent important traditional practices for some patients and their families.[7] Respect for such cultural practices, with creation of a safe clinical environment for their disclosure, consideration of how they link to patient's cultural/spiritual/religious values, and evaluation of their role in the patient's care, is an important part of respecting the autonomy of patients and families and establishing and maintaining therapeutic alliance.[7] The growing use of CAM combined with limited standardization of ingredients within natural products, little oversight by regulatory bodies such as the FDA, and lacking evidence for their efficacy or safety, pose challenges for their use within Western medical contexts.[20] Medical providers must balance ethical duties to respect patient and family care preferences for the use of herbal products, whose use may also be beneficent through respecting patient wishes and potential benefits from plant-based remedies, with nonmaleficence and the potential for harm, as herbal products could potentially pose harms through unknown actions, adverse effects, and drug interactions.[20]

To meet ethical obligations to promote patient welfare, through respecting patient and family stated preferences and providing effective medical treatment with reduction of potential harms, psychiatric prescribers have a duty to become familiar with CAM, assess for CAM in routine clinical assessments, and research the natural products used by their patients, with pharmacy consultation as needed.[20] To effectively evaluate the risks and benefits of CAM, providers are encouraged to consider the following: (1) Acuity, severity, and prognosis of the medical or psychiatric condition; (2) efficacy and adverse effects of conventional medical treatments; (3) quality of evidence, efficacy, and safety profile of CAM; (4) patient/family understanding of the risk-benefit profile of CAM treatment; and (5) importance, persistence, and rationale for patient/family values to use CAM.[7,20] When evaluation and research regarding CAM interventions demonstrate evidence for their safety and efficacy, duties to autonomy, beneficence, and nonmaleficence are aligned, and it is ethically permissible to support patient use of CAM.[7] For CAM that has concerning evidence that it may be unsafe and harmful to patients, the principle of nonmaleficence requires that practitioners inform the patient of potential harms and work with the patient/family, and as feasible, their CAM prescriber, to support the integration of safer CAM practices into their care.[7] Finally, as in the case of Mr L, when there is lacking evidence regarding CAM safety and efficacy, practitioners are encouraged to review the lack of data for the safety and efficacy of the proposed CAM treatment with patients and families.[7] Providers may consider close monitoring of the CAM treatment with the physician and herbalist and alternate CAM natural products with more robust evidence or within the mind/body practice realm and/or a trial off of the CAM intervention and monitor clinical symptoms.[7] For Mr L, given strong patient and family preferences to continue CAM with tolerability over the week, in the absence of adverse effect, the decision was made to continue his complementary treatment with ongoing close monitoring and involvement of his herbalist in his ongoing care.

Clinical Vignette

On your final evaluation with Mr L and his wife and daughter, before hospital discharge, they note being very pleased with the consistent use of Mandarin interpretation services as well as integration of their herbalist into Mr L's medical care. Mr L discusses feeling that the prescribed antidepressant medication has aided in returning energy flow to his mind and body and that he is amenable to continue to engage with you for outpatient monitoring of his mood symptoms and antidepressant therapy. They note that this has been a positive care experience, in contrast to prior hospitalizations, where they have experienced communication barriers and limited ability to disclose their care concerns and have them be acknowledged in the care setting.

Patient Autonomy and Promotion of Accessible Culturally Competent Care

Recognizing culture's influence on social norms is important for understanding behaviors that might be representative of illness or functional impairment, explanatory models of behavioral concerns, preferred treatment modalities, and help-seeking behaviors.[21] The strong Western cultural influence on the mental health field, with continued emphasis on mind-body duality and the locus of psychiatric pathologic condition within the individual, rather than the family or community, may be incompatible with culturally diverse approaches to behavioral concerns.[21] Despite efforts to broaden cultural awareness and understanding in relation to illness, such as the DSM-5 cultural formulation, barriers continue to challenge the integration of multicultural views within mental health treatment paradigms and the provision of equitable, accessible mental health care services across cultural and ethnic minorities.[21] Appeals to principles of distributive justice further highlight the ethical duties to ensure persons from diverse cultural communities have equitable access to mental health services, with efforts to reduce and ameliorate persistent disparities.[7]

Existing challenges in the engagement of culturally diverse populations in mental health care may relate to stigma, racism and discrimination, and patient-provider power inequities.[21] Stigma related to behavioral symptoms or diagnosis of mental health challenges may be linked to concern with the need to protect personal dignity and familial reputation, and fear of being harshly judged or misunderstood by clinicians, with potential for loss of control and involuntary treatment.[21] The pervasive nature of racism and discrimination within Western society toward minority ethnic and cultural groups, particularly among cultural groups with histories of oppression and intergenerational trauma, can lead to mistrust toward Western medical providers, out of fear of the potential for being stereotyped, inaccurately diagnosed or overpathologized, with inappropriate or inadequate care, in the medical setting.[21] The patient-provider relationship also faces additional challenges in a multicultural care context, with potential for power-differentials based on dominant and minority cultural affiliations, language and communication challenges, and poor family involvement in care.[21] Such factors have the potential to reduce patient autonomy if care is experienced as misaligned with their cultural beliefs and values.[21]

Potential solutions to address these care barriers and promote equitable mental health care access for minority groups may include efforts to reduce stigma through integrated behavioral health models, where psychiatric care can be accessed within the medical context, as well as integration of mental health services within more culturally attuned and accessible community-based clinics.[21] Fostering cultural partnerships between mental health care providers and community cultural leaders, such as religious practitioners and traditional healers, may assist in reduction of stigma, discrimination, and power-differentials and promote mental health education and engagement.[21] Continued promotion of cultural competence and humility training with use of standardized cultural assessment tools in mental health evaluation is critical to continue to promote provision of mental health care service engagement across culturally diverse patient populations. Continued advocacy efforts are needed to foster awareness and funding for policy changes to promote culturally competent and equitable care across the United States, given the increasing population diversity and growing need for multicultural approaches in mental health care settings.

SUMMARY

Promotion of cultural competence in mental health care has emerged to respect the diversity of patient values and care preferences to enhance patient engagement and the quality of their medical care. Patients from diverse cultures may prefer non-Western models of care, and providers must be aware and able to accommodate, diverse care models, including those adopting relational autonomy standards with close familial involvement to navigate clinical care choices. Given the growing cultural diversity within United States care settings, continued efforts to promote care attuned to cultural diversity are needed to address existing barriers for minority populations and promote equitable care access across all cultures and ethnicities.

DISCLOSURE STATEMENT

The author has nothing to disclose.

REFERENCES

1. American Psychiatric Association. APA commentary on ethics in practice. 2015. Available at: https://www.psychiatry.org/file%20library/psychiatrists/practice/ethics/apa-commentary-on-ethics-in-practice.pdf. Accessed August 9, 2021.
2. Beauchamp TL, Childress JF. Principles of biomedical ethics. 7th edition. New York: Oxford University Press; 2013.
3. Spatz ES, Krumholz HM, Moulton BW. The new era of informed consent. Getting to a reasonable-patient standard through shared decision making. JAMA 2016; 315(19):2063–4.
4. Turoldo F. Relational autonomy and multiculturalism. Dissection bioethics. Camb Q HealthC Ethics 2010;19:542–9.
5. Blackhall LJ, Murphy ST, Frank G, et al. Ethnicity and attitudes toward patient autonomy. JAMA 1995;274(10):820–5.
6. Fu-Chang Tsia D. Personhood and autonomy in multicultural health care settings. Virtual Mentor 2008;10(3):171–6.
7. Hoop JG, DiPasquale T, Hernandez JM, et al. Ethics and culture in mental health care. Ethics Behav 2008;18(4):353–72.
8. American Psychiatric Association. The diagnostic and statistical manual. 5th edition. Washington, DC: American Psychiatric Publishing; 2013.
9. Stubbe D. Practicing cultural competence and cultural humility in the care of diverse patients. Focus 2020;18(1):49–51. Available at: https://focus.psychiatryonline.org/doi/pdf/10.1176/appi.focus.20190041.
10. Hwang W, Myers HF, Abe-Kim J, et al. A conceptual paradigm for understanding culture's impact on mental health: the cultural influences on mental health (CIMH) model. Clin Psychol Rev 2008;28:211–27.
11. McGuire TG, Miranda J. Racial and ethnic disparities in mental health care: evidence and policy implications. Health Aff (Millwood) 2008;27(2):393–403.
12. Timmons M. Moral theory: an introduction. 2nd edition. Lanham, MD: Rowman & Littlefield; 2013.
13. Knapp S. When values of different cultures conflict: ethical decision making in a multicultural context. Prof Psychol Res Pract 2007;38(6):660–6.
14. Ho A. Relational autonomy or undue pressure? Family's role in medical decision-making. Scand J Caring Sci 2008;22:128–35.

15. Yeung A. Ethical and cultural considerations in delivering psychiatric diagnosis: reconciling the gap using MDD diagnosis and delivery in less acculturated Chinese patients. Transcult Psychiatry 2008;45(4):531–52.
16. Chettih M. Turning the lens inward: cultural competence and providers' values in health care decision making. Gerontologist 2012;52(6):739–47.
17. Appelbaum P. Assessment of patients' competence to consent to treatment. N Engl J Med 2007;357:1834–40.
18. Waldfogel S, Measows S. Religious issues in the capacity evaluation. Gen Hosp Psychiatry 1996;18:173–82.
19. Sedig L. What's the role of autonomy in patient-and-family-centered care when patients and family member's don't agree. Am Med Assoc J Ethics 2016; 18(1):12–7.
20. Krause B, Lavretsky H, Dunn LB, et al. Ethical challenges in complementary and alternative medicine. Focus 2018;16(1):63–6.
21. Gopalkrishnan N. Cultural diversity and mental health: considerations for policy and practice. Front Public Health 2018;6(179):1–7.

Practical Research Ethics in Psychiatric Clinical Trials
A Guide for Investigators

Michelle Hume, MD, PhD[a],*, Melissa Abraham, PhD, MSc[b,c,d,e]

KEYWORDS

- Ethics • Psychiatric research • Clinical research • Human subjects
- Mental illness research • Institutional review board

KEY POINTS

- The current clinical standard of care is typically used as the ethical gold standard by which the diagnostic and therapeutic treatments in a psychiatric research study are judged.
- Critically important in psychiatric research is that the law in most US jurisdictions requires confidential treatment of adolescents for mental health, substance use, and reproductive health.
- There is a paucity of research on psychiatric inpatients, but Institutional Review Boards frequently require additional protections when enrolling patients who are psychiatrically hospitalized.
- Despite efforts by the National Institutes of Health (NIH) to require NIH-funded clinical trials to include women and minorities as participants and to assess outcomes by sex and race or ethnicity, studies over time have found no changes in inclusion, analysis, or reporting.
- When sensitive information such as criminal behavior, sexual abuse history, legal history, and illicit drug use is collected for research, extra precautions to protect both privacy and confidentiality are indicated.

INTRODUCTION

The conduct of clinical psychiatric research is critical to ensure that safe and effective therapies are adequately tested in populations representative of those in whom they will be used, to strengthen our systems of care, and to enhance our ability to advance and deliver care effectively to patients regardless of race, gender, or ethnicity. There are unique ethical considerations regarding the conduct of research involving patients with mental illness, due to variable impacts on cognition and decisional capacity, stigma

[a] Mendota Mental Health Institute, 301 Troy Dr, Madison, WI 53704, USA; [b] Research Ethics Consultation Unit, Division of Clinical Research, Massachusetts General Hospital; [c] Department of Psychiatry, Massachusetts General Hospital, Harvard Medical School; [d] Center for Bioethics, Harvard Medical School; [e] Ariadne Labs
* Corresponding author.
E-mail address: Michelle.Hume@dhs.wisconsin.gov

Psychiatr Clin N Am 44 (2021) 549–561
https://doi.org/10.1016/j.psc.2021.08.005

associated with having mental illness, and diminished social influence related to mental illness. A detailed review of the development of research ethics guidelines underlying the conduct of psychiatric research has been conducted extensively elsewhere.[1,2]

From a regulatory standpoint, Federal regulations governing research on humans at 45 CFR 46 and 21 CFR 50 require Institutional Review Boards (IRBs) to review research according to a specific set of criteria in order to approve the research. Regulations require IRBs to consist of members with varying backgrounds who have the professional competence necessary to conduct an ethical and regulatory review of proposed research activities, as well as members sensitive to the rights and welfare of members of diverse populations who may participate in research [see 45 CFR 46.108(b), 21 CFR 56.108(c)]. In general terms, IRB must ensure that risks to participants are minimized, risks are reasonable in relation to the anticipated benefits of the research and the importance of the knowledge that is expected to result, selection of participants is equitable, adequate provisions are made for consent, data are monitored to ensure the safety of participants, and that privacy and confidentiality of research participants is protected. Although federal regulations provide explicit additional protections for participants from some vulnerable populations such and children and prisoners, there are no explicit protections in the regulations for members of other potentially vulnerable groups, such as the elderly or the mentally ill, despite these groups' and individuals' potential vulnerability due to traits such as impaired decision-making capacity or increased reliance on family or caregivers.

Investigators wishing for a primer on medical ethics are directed to the classic textbook by Beauchamp and Childress, Principles of Biomedical Ethics.[3] In this text, the investigators discuss in detail the 4 principles of Respect for Autonomy, Nonmaleficence, Beneficence, and Justice. They comment as well on the distinction between clinical and research ethics and address ethical considerations arising in particular for members of vulnerable populations. With respect to research ethics specifically, Emanuel and colleagues' article outlining 7 requirements necessary for ethical clinical research provides an important overview.[4] In summary, clinical research must be valuable, have scientific validity, equitable subject selection, a favorable risk-benefit profile, have independent review, informed consent, and respect for potential and enrolled participants.[4]

The perspective herein emerges from the investigators' positions in which investigators wanting to perform clinical research with individuals with psychiatric conditions have sought practical advice on how to conduct their research in an ethical manner and on issues that may be of concern to research ethics authorities. The intent of this article is, therefore, to provide (1) an overview of common ethical considerations when conducting psychiatric clinical research, along with (2) practical advice for preparing IRB applications and associated materials. Where appropriate, the authors also include references to applicable Food and Drug Administration (FDA) guidance. A full list of FDA guidance documents pertaining to clinical trials is available at https://www.fda.gov/regulatory-information/search-fda-guidance-documents/clinical-trials-guidance-documents. These documents may serve as a useful starting point or reference regarding the research landscape, regardless of whether the study is formally FDA regulated.

The following key points of particular relevance in psychiatric clinical research are now addressed in the coming sections of this article:

1. Appropriate Protection of Placebo Control Groups
2. Therapeutic Misconception
3. Pediatric Psychiatric Clinical Research
4. Capacity to Provide Informed Consent

5. Research on Hospitalized Patients
6. Inclusion of Underrepresented Minorities in Clinical Psychiatric Research, and
7. Privacy and Confidentiality.

DISCUSSION OF KEY POINTS
Appropriate Protection of Placebo Control Groups

In psychiatry, placebo-controlled studies are often the most efficient design and easiest to interpret and as such are frequently preferred by industry for pivotal registrational studies.[5] In circumstances in which a placebo is necessary to answer the research question, IRBs review protections for patients in the control group especially carefully, consistent with risk minimization requirements. The current clinical standard of care is typically used as the ethical gold standard by which the diagnostic and therapeutic treatments in the study are judged. Sometimes, but not always, IRBs will consider local factors as well, such as the availability of treatments or providers in the local area outside of the study when assessing standard of care. As such, investigators should think carefully about how procedures in the proposed study, including using a placebo arm itself, deviate from clinical standards of care in ways that may place participants at risk.

Some psychotropic drug trials include a period before randomization in which all participants receive placebo. Depending on the purpose, these periods are referred to as "washout" periods during which any prestudy medications are stopped, or "run-in" periods in which all participants are given placebo as a means of eliminating placebo responders or nonadherent participants from later randomization, ensuring that participants are stable, or simply to provide a period for baseline measurement. The practice is common in psychotropic drug studies[6] and are often single-blind, meaning that investigators, but not participants, are aware that participants are receiving placebo during this phase. However, the evidence for the statistical utility of run-in periods in psychiatric drug studies is mixed at best.[7–14] The ethical concern involves deception,[15,16] either that this period is not mentioned at all in standard consent forms or that the "disclosure" is couched in highly general language about the possibility that any participant could receive placebo. Given these factors, ethical considerations argue in favor of investigators considering single-blind treatment periods either disclosing them openly in consent documents or requesting consultation with their local IRB regarding what is permissible locally, even if not most ethical.

A second potential concern about placebo run-in designs is disruption in care. When run-in periods are relatively short and are followed by the initiation of an appropriate active medication in a stable study population, the IRB may find the study design relatively unproblematic due to limited likely effect of medication discontinuation. However, if the run-in period is followed by randomization to placebo, a participant may end up off medication for a much longer period. As such, the key ethical issue is whether the duration of placebo exposure is justifiable in members of the population that is enrolled in the study and/or whether there are additional treatments that are permitted in the placebo group to mitigate the risks of medication discontinuation.

Although monitoring of participant safety is critical in any trial, increased monitoring may partially alleviate concerns related to psychiatric clinical trials with placebo exposure. One approach is monitoring participants for symptom emergence and exacerbation more frequently than would be performed in standard treatment settings. Included in this monitoring approach is the requirement for prospective assessments of emergent suicidal ideation and behavior in all FDA-regulated studies of products being developed for any psychiatric indication, antiepileptic drugs, or any drug with central nervous system activity. The FDA guidance on this topic is extensive and covers agency requirements in a variety of settings.[17] The bottom line is that clear criteria should be delineated for withdrawing participants promptly from a study due to worsening symptoms out of respect for persons and obligations not to harm (nonmaleficence). Finally, investigators will need to explain how excluded study participants (particularly those with exacerbation of psychiatric symptoms) will be referred for timely and appropriate care outside of the study in accordance with ethical principles of helping (beneficence), avoiding harm (nonmaleficence), and fair allocation of resources (justice).

Therapeutic Misconception

In 1982, Appelbaum and colleagues reported interviews with psychiatric patients documenting failure to appreciate the difference between research and treatment and labeled the phenomenon "therapeutic misconception."[18] A later consensus definition opined that "therapeutic misconception exists when individuals do not understand that the defining purpose of clinical research is to produce generalizable knowledge, regardless of whether the subjects enrolled in the trial may potentially benefit from the intervention under study or from other aspects of the clinical trial."[19] In particular, participants should understand the uncertainty regarding risks and benefits of the investigational intervention, that there may be interventions or procedures that are not clinically necessary, the adherence to a protocol rather than individual clinician judgment, and the clinician's role as an investigator. It is the responsibility of the researcher/clinician to be sure the potential participant understands the difference between treatment and research and to outline how this will be communicated and appreciated in the recruitment and informed consent details of the research protocol. These measures are ethically important in consideration of respect for persons and their rational decision-making (respect for autonomy), to avoid coercion and lack of informed consent that erode autonomy, and obligations to refrain from causing harm (nonmaleficence).

Recent empirical reviews suggest that therapeutic misconception in psychiatric research continues to be common.[20] Interventions to reduce therapeutic misconception may include the use of neutral educators who have no affiliation with the research project to disclose information to potential participants and the provision of financial compensation to impress on subjects that they are providing a social service by volunteering for clinical research, although the amount must be carefully determined to avoid potential coercion. Enhanced educational interventions that augment typical informed consent have specifically been shown to reduced therapeutic misconception in a randomized trial.[21] Overall, to respect the interests of and fulfill responsibilities to research participants, the consent process optimally should clearly delineate procedures that are done for research purposes only and pay particular attention to how research and benefit is explained. For patients who may fluctuate in their ability to engage in the informed consent process, investigators should be mindful that consent is a process rather than an event and that ongoing assessment of consent and capacity may be ethically warranted, especially in research participants who are vulnerable and/or cognitively impaired.

Both undue inducement and therapeutic misconception may be substantial concerns when potential research participants lack access to timely or appropriate psychiatric care. For example, suppose a patient who meets criteria for major depression came to the emergency department of a medical center conducting a research study on treatments for major depressive disorder. The patient might be either put on a months-long wait list to see a mental health clinician or be offered a screening visit for a research study within 1 to 2 days. In these situations, IRBs may limit the financial remuneration to participants as undue inducement and pay careful attention to evaluate communications in resource-scarce recruitment settings out of concerns of potential undue inducement/coercion, beneficence, nonmaleficence, and justice. At times, IRBs may also require scripted language for investigators to follow regarding how a study is presented to potential participants.

Pediatrics

The historical dearth of information on drugs labeled for pediatric use led to children being called therapeutic orphans, for whom most drugs were prescribed off-label. In 1975, only 22% of drugs were adequately labeled for pediatric use.[22] Research on children is typically not cost-effective for the pharmaceutical industry because of the low expected market share of most pediatric indications. Subsequent legislation and regulations both incentivizing and requiring pediatric studies have led to increased labeling of new products for pediatric use.[23] NIH also recently created a pediatric research consortium to harmonize and set priorities across NIH-funded pediatric studies.[24]

Additional protections for children in clinical research exist in both HHS and FDA regulations in recognition of the responsibilities for well-being of minors (beneficence and nonmaleficence), their ongoing growth and development, and respecting personhood while avoiding disproportionate burden. In general, these ethical considerations are expressed through regulations that limit the degree of acceptable risk in pediatric research that does not offer potential medical benefit to enrolled children and contain provisions for parental permission and child assent. Whether permission is required from one or both parents depends on the category of research under which the study is approved by the local IRB. If the study is considered minimal risk (45 CFR 46.404 and 21 CFR 50.51) or has the prospect of providing direct medical benefit (45 CFR 45.405 and 21 CFR 50.52) for the enrolled child, the permission of one parent is sufficient. For research that is judged to be greater than minimal risk and is without direct benefit to the child, permission generally must be obtained from both parents in recognition of the importance and seriousness of informed consent and the interest of the child in settings of potential harm and no reciprocal direct benefit. Guidance on obtaining permission when both parents are not reasonably available was recently published by the Secretary's Advisory Committee on Human Research Protections.[25] In all categories of research, the assent of enrolled children is required in recognition of their personhood notwithstanding developmental and chronologic age limitations in the ability to formally participate in and give full informed consent (see later discussion). As such, federal guidance suggests that assent should be obtained from children 6 years of age and older. Most IRBs recommend making separate assent documents for younger children (eg, ages 6–11 years) and adolescents.

Critically important in psychiatric research is that respect for persons and the prevention of harm is codified in state law in most places to, inter alia, require confidential treatment of adolescents for mental health, substance use, and reproductive health. Whether such treatment statutes extend to research participation depends on the interpretation of the law in the local jurisdiction in which the research is conducted. As such, investigators have a responsibility to keep abreast of this information. In the authors' experience, most institutions, in accordance with ethical principles and prevailing legal protections for sensitive health information, interpret the law in favor of adolescent confidentiality. If so, then although parental consent is required for initial participation in the study, investigators then have a responsibility to keep information regarding mental health and pregnancy confidential from parents if requested by adolescents. Legal consultation within one's institution is often warranted, and IRBs often have standard language and procedures related to confi-dentiality and minors.

Another area of controversy is the use of placebo controls in medication trials involving children. The FDA has adopted the position that the risk-benefit profiles of interventions or procedures should be assessed individually rather than collectively.[26] From an ethics standpoint, protection of children and adolescents as members of a vulnerable popula-tion informs this regulatory policy. As such, the placebo arm of a pediatric study must not exceed a minor increase over minimal risk. "For such a trial to be approvable by a local IRB under 21 CFR part 50, subpart D, the risk to children randomized to a comparator group that involves the withholding of…treatment (whether placebo or delayed therapy) must be no more than a minor increase over minimal risk (21 CFR 50.53). In addition, clin-ical trials must be designed so that risks to patients are minimized (21 CFR 56.111)."[27] Although there is no formal guidance on the degree of risk acceptable as a minor increase over minimal risk, and interpretation of the standard is variable among IRB chairs. Many, but not all, IRB chairs considered allergy skin testing to be a minor increase over minimal risk, as well as MRIs without the use of procedural sedation. Investigators considering the use of placebo controls in children should consult their local IRB for a determination regarding the acceptability of their proposed research.[28] Further ethical attention and exploration may be used to hone approaches to the factors to be considered in determi-nations of what constitutes minimal versus more than minimal risk.

Capacity to Provide Informed Consent

The foundational principle of informed consent is autonomy, which "encompasses at a minimum, self-rule that is, free from both controlling interference by others and from certain limitations such as an inadequate understanding that prevents meaningful choice."[3] Informed consent also requires having adequate information about the risks, benefits, and alternatives to make an appropriate decision about whether study partic-ipation is in accordance with one's interests and desires. As noted earlier, both med-ical and psychiatric conditions have the potential to lead to impaired capacity to consent. However, due primarily to issues of stigma around mental illness, impaired consent capacity has become strongly associated with psychiatric illness. Although it is certainly true that severely ill persons may have impaired capacity to consent while acutely ill, the same may be true of patients with a variety of serious nonpsychiatric illnesses. As with any research participant, psychiatric patients with impaired capacity should be routinely reassessed to see if they have regained capacity.

There are a variety of ways to assess capacity when needed in clinical research. One of the most common is The MacArthur Competency Assessment Tool-Clinical Research (MacCAT-CR), which was adapted in 2001 from a semistructured interview developed for use in medical treatment contexts.[29] The MacCAT-CR combines infor-mation disclosure with a capacity assessment to consent to clinical research and can be performed in approximately 15 minutes. Using this instrument, even potential research participants with acute psychosis may be able to provide informed con-sent.[30] Briefer screening tools have also been developed that are intended to help in-vestigators identify research participants who warrant more thorough decisional capacity assessment and/or remediation efforts before enrollment.[31] Shorter clinical screening tests such as the Mini-Mental Status Examination are at best mediocre pre-dictors of capacity as measured by the MacCAT-CR.[32]

Research on Hospitalized Patients

Due in part to ethical concerns about the appropriateness of enrolling severely ill indi-viduals in placebo-controlled studies of psychotropic medication, typical efficacy studies of psychotropic medications are poorly generalizable. Reviews of treatment trials of antidepressants,[33] agents for bipolar disorder,[34] personality disorders,[35] and substance use disorders[36] uniformly conclude that the overwhelming majority of typical clinical populations with each disorder would be excluded. In particular, there is a paucity of research on psychiatric inpatients, who are often considered highly vulnerable due to the acuity of their symptoms and the possibility of impaired capacity to consent. In these circumstances, consent may be impaired both due to symptoms and due to confinement in a locked inpatient psychiatric unit, as addressed in further discussion.

The inclusion of psychiatric inpatients in research rests in the federal regulations on the requirement for equitable selection of subjects, found at (45 CFR 46.111[3]). In making this assessment, the IRB considers the purposes of the research and the setting in which the research will be conducted. From a practical perspective, the IRB will assess whether the target population is appropriate to answer the research question, whether any individuals are being excluded from a study or being targeted for inclusion without sufficient justification, and whether the research will benefit the proposed subject population.

Although involuntary psychiatric patients admitted to nonpenal facilities do not meet the regulatory definition of prisoners, they are frequently confined to a facility against their will that they do not have the freedom to leave and in which patients may perceive that "good behavior" may influence the length of their stay. In this regard, there are important ethical parallels between psychiatric inpatients and persons in legal custody such as prisoners, and IRBs may reasonably require additional protections of research enrolling psychiatric inpatients. At a minimum, they may require that such research directly relate to the patient's condition as a psychiatric inpatient (eg, could not be carried out on psychiatric outpatients) or place constraints around the degree of risk that is allowable. These measures address the important ethical considerations of autonomy, beneficence, nonmaleficence, and justice by addressing protection of the individual's bodily integrity, advancing care and limiting harm, and avoiding both disproportionate burden and lack of access to clinical study.

In 2018, the American Psychiatric Association published a Position Statement on Research with Involuntary Psychiatric Patients,[37] similarly concluding that "hospitalized psychiatric patients, including those who are involuntarily committed, should be permitted to participate in research, so long as appropriate safeguards are in place; and consistent with respect for their autonomy, patients are able to exercise adequate informed consent." However, institutions may also be wary of public perception of such studies; the Department of Veteran's Affairs Office of the Inspector General called the recent enrollment of an involuntary patient in a research study "ethically questionable" because of concerns that the patient may have conflated the voluntary nature of research participation with the involuntary nature of the mental health commitment.[38]

Prior research indicates that perceived coercion for psychiatric treatment or civil commitment is not related to voluntary or involuntary status in any straightforward way. In one study, about 10% of voluntary patients felt coerced into admission and 35% of involuntary patients did not feel coerced.[39] In addition to prominently highlighting in consent documents that participation will not affect the length of hospitalization or any court proceedings (if applicable), investigators may wish to consider additional protections as well. Provided patients are agreeable, the intentional involvement of family members in discussions about research participation is one measure to reduce the appearance of and/or perceived/experienced coercion. There is continued tension in this area, with some institutions avoiding enrollment of individuals in research during the initial involuntary phase (~3 days, depending on state law) for both legal and ethical reasons, whereas others highlight some of the need to study this crucial period of illness.

Inclusion of Underrepresented Minorities

The lack of inclusion of women and nonwhite populations in medical research continues to be an area of concern. Medical experimentation on African Americans during slavery[40] as well as in the infamous US Public Health Service's Tuskegee Study of Untreated Syphilis in the Male Negro laid a foundation of mistrust toward health care providers.[41] Further, studies have shown that Black patients continue to receive fewer appropriate mental health services than comparable white populations and may be more likely to receive stigmatizing diagnoses based on race.[42,43] Despite efforts to require NIH-funded clinical trials to include women and minorities as participants and assess outcomes by sex and race or ethnicity, studies over time have found no changes in inclusion, analysis, or reporting.[44] As such, merely passive efforts to recruit sufficient minorities into research are unlikely to successfully recruit a representative population.

As in clinical contexts, conducting research with underrepresented populations requires sustained outreach and building of trust with underserved communities. It is important for clinicians to acknowledge psychosocial stressors that may be unique to minoritized populations, including their experience with systemic racism. Allowing extra time for participants to fully explore any reservations about treatment or participation is also crucial. In addition, inquiring about social support networks and religious or spiritual involvement or affiliation and, with permission, encouraging potential study participants to seek input from other trusted individuals may improve trust and ultimately participation in research. Providers must recognize, however, that collateral parties may be strategic allies or, alternatively, barriers to research intervention.

Protocols and IRB applications should clearly outline minority enrollment targets and detail specific plans for increasing minority enrollment to continue to advance research equity. The National Cancer Institute created a successful grant program by building clinical trials outreach and management capacity in health care institutions serving large numbers of minority patients.[45] Similar efforts in other areas have demonstrated the need to establish a presence and approach underrepresented communities in the places that they commonly seek care.

Privacy and Confidentiality

When sensitive information such as criminal behavior, sexual abuse history, legal history, and illicit drug use is collected for research, extra precautions to protect both privacy and confidentiality are warranted grounded in ethical commitments to respecting participants. Privacy generally refers to an individual's right to control access to their personal information, which may include health conditions. Issues such as subject selection, recruitment strategies, and data collection methods are particularly important to consider. Confidentiality typically refers to how private information provided by individuals will be protected by researchers from release. Investigators must both demonstrate their understanding of both concepts to IRBs and take appropriate measures to minimize risks. In particular, the need to collect sensitive information must be clearly justified in the protocol. Detail should be provided in both the protocol and the informed consent document regarding how such information will be collected, transmitted, recorded, and stored. The very fact of participation in a study with a title indicating a psychiatric condition can be a breach of confidentiality, and institutions vary in their approach to minimizing this risk. Investigators should therefore be aware of their ethical responsibilities to participants in designing and implementing clinical trials.

As is true in psychiatric care, information disclosed within a research context may be subject to reporting requirements or may entail that a potential subject would be referred for voluntary or involuntary psychiatric treatment outside of the study. In addition, at times, investigators may wish to review the participants' psychiatric records as part of the investigation. Should this be true, investigators must inform participants of what information will be reviewed and recorded within the research record, as such information is also subject to review by federal regulatory entities. As such, absolute privacy and confidentiality cannot be guaranteed. From an ethics standpoint, these exceptions to confidentiality serve important public health and regulatory purposes justifying the deprioritization of the individual's privacy in favor of the public good. Although Certificates of Confidentiality (COCs) may seem to override state law reporting requirements, in general this question has remained untested in state courts, and many research institutions will voluntarily comply regardless. Further, COCs do not protect against voluntary disclosures by research subjects and do not protect participants against federal audit of research records.

With respect to privacy, consideration should be given for the cultural norms and ages of the participant population, as privacy concerns may differ. Investigators should also be thoughtful about how potential participants will be identified and approached. It is generally not acceptable to have a member of the research team who has had no prior contact with a patient approach or contact potential participants, unless those individuals have given permission to be contacted. With respect to the method of data collection, consideration needs to be given to the sensitivity of the information being collected and whether a private interview setting is needed.

The level of safeguards needed to ensure confidentiality of participants' private information may vary considerably between studies. However, it is important to remember that even studies that pose no physical risks to participants may collect highly sensitive information that poses significant risk to participants' privacy, insurability, employability if disclosed. For example, an international consortium recently described 109 genetic variants associated with 8 psychiatric disorders: autism, attention-deficit hyperactivity disorder, schizophrenia, bipolar disorder, depression, obsessive-compulsive disorder, and Tourette syndrome, in a total of about 230,000 patients worldwide.[46] As such, these studies may require relatively robust multilevel systems to ensure data confidentiality, even if the study merely collects genetic information.

SUMMARY

In this article, the authors have reviewed key ethical considerations for investigators wishing to conduct psychiatric research: appropriate protection of placebo control groups, therapeutic misconception, pediatrics, capacity to provide informed consent, research on hospitalized patients, inclusion of underrepresented minorities, and privacy and confidentiality. Once investigators have considered each of these issues carefully, the final task is to create a high-quality IRB application to support the proposed research. Investigators should not assume that IRBs understand nuances of clinical care of psychiatric conditions or necessarily what standard of care treatment may involve for participants outside of the proposed research study. Given that many benefit-risk determinations regarding study participation hinge on care that is available outside of the study, good-quality IRB applications typically provide a brief explanation of standard of care. Where possible, empirical and clinical support should be provided for approaches to controversial questions. Finally, having experienced clinicians and researchers involved in a supervisory capacity and detailing plans for supervision of younger team members may be reassuring to ethics review committees.

DISCLOSURE

Neither of the authors have any commercial or financial conflicts of interest, and no dedicated funding was received for this article.

REFERENCES

1. Barry LK. Ethical issues in psychiatric research. Psychiatr Clin North Am 2009; 32(2):381–94.
2. Tsao CI, Layde JB, Roberts LW. A review of ethics in psychiatric research. Curr Opin Psychiatry 2008;21(6):572–7.
3. Beauchamp TL. Principles of biomedical ethics. 8th edition. New York, NY: Oxford University Press; 2019.
4. Emanuel EJ, Wendler D, Grady C. What makes clinical research ethical? JAMA 2000;283(20):2701–11.
5. Food and Drug Administration. Guidance for industry E 10 choice of control group and related issues in clinical trials. 2001. Available at: https://www.fda.gov/media/71349/download. Accessed September 17, 2021.
6. Chen YF, Yang Y, Hung HM, et al. Evaluation of performance of some enrichment designs dealing with high placebo response in psychiatric clinical trials. Contemp Clin Trials 2011;32(4):592–604.
7. Bridge JA, Iyengar S, Salary CB, et al. Clinical response and risk for reported suicidal ideation and suicide attempts in pediatric antidepressant treatment: a meta-analysis of randomized controlled trials. JAMA 2007;297(15):1683–96.
8. Khan A, Cohen S, Dager S, et al. Onset of response in relation to outcome in depressed outpatients with placebo and imipramine. J Affect Disord 1989; 17(1):33–8.
9. Trivedi MH, Rush H. Does a placebo run-in or a placebo treatment cell affect the efficacy of antidepressant medications? Neuropsychopharmacology 1994;11(1): 33–43.
10. Lee S, Walker JR, Jakul L, et al. Does elimination of placebo responders in a placebo run-in increase the treatment effect in randomized clinical trials? A meta-analytic evaluation. Depress Anxiety 2004;19(1):10–9.
11. Greenberg RP, Fisher S, Riter JA. Placebo washout is not a meaningful part of antidepressant drug trials. Percept Mot Skills 1995;81(2):688–90.
12. Mitte K, Noack P, Steil R, et al. A meta-analytic review of the efficacy of drug treatment in generalized anxiety disorder. J Clin Psychopharmacol 2005;25(2):141–50.
13. Del Re AC, Maisel N, Blodgett J, et al. The declining efficacy of naltrexone pharmacotherapy for alcohol use disorders over time: a multivariate meta-analysis. Alcohol Clin Exp Res 2013;37(6):1064–8.
14. Hulshof TA, Zuidema SU, Gispen-de Wied CC, et al. Run-in periods and clinical outcomes of antipsychotics in dementia: a meta-epidemiological study of placebo-controlled trials. Pharmacoepidemiol Drug Saf 2020;29(2):125–33.
15. Kukla R. Resituating the principle of equipoise: justice and access to care in non-ideal conditions. Kennedy Inst Ethics J 2007;17(3):171–202.
16. Senn S. Are placebo run ins justified? BMJ 1997;314(7088):1191–3.
17. Food and Drug Administration. Guidance for industry: suicidal ideation and behavior: prospective assessment of occurrence in clinical trials. 2012. Available

at: https://nam11.safelinks.protection.outlook.com/?url=https%3A%2F%2Fwww.fda.gov%2Fregulatory-information%2Fsearch-fda-guidance-documents%2Fguidance-industry-suicidal-ideation-and-behavior-prospective-assessment-occurrence-clinical-trials&data=04%7C01%7Cm.packiam%40elsevier.com%7Cc8e86e3441824dfc3dc508d97a0b4f77%7C9274ee3f94254109a27f9fb15c10675d%7C0%7C0%7C637675011657758073%7CUnknown%7CTWFpbGZsb3d8eyJWIjoiMC4wLjAwMDAiLCJQIjoiV2luMzIiLCJBTiI6Ik1haWwiLCJXVCI6Mn0%3D%7C3000&sdata=%2FByy1dJnJ4Dyupcxo8SE%2BSd2ncoTsWo%2F46pWBwUn8uc%3D&reserved=0. Accessed September 17, 2021.

18. Appelbaum PS, Roth LH, Lidz C. The therapeutic misconception: informed consent in psychiatric research. Int J Law Psychiatry 1982;5(3–4):319–29.

19. Henderson GE, Churchill LR, Davis AM, et al. Clinical trials and medical care: defining the therapeutic misconception. PLoS Med 2007;4(11):e324.

20. Thong IS, Foo MY, Sum MY, et al. Therapeutic misconception in psychiatry research: a systematic review. Clin Psychopharmacol Neurosci 2016;14(1):17–25.

21. Christopher PP, Appelbaum PS, Truong D, et al. Reducing therapeutic misconception: a randomized intervention trial in hypothetical clinical trials. PLoS One 2017;12(9):e0184224.

22. Wilson JT. Pragmatic assessment of medicines available for young children and pregnant or breast-feeding women. In: Basic and therapeutic aspects of perinatal pharmacology. New York, NY: Raven Press; 1975. p. 411–21.

23. Sachs AN, Avant D, Lee CS, et al. Pediatric information in drug product labeling. JAMA 2012;307(18):1914–5.

24. New trans-NIH consortium aims to advance pediatric research on a global level. 2018. Available at: https://www.nichd.nih.gov/newsroom/news/061318-trans-NIH-consortium. Accessed July 1, 2020.

25. Secretary's Advisory Committee for Human Research Protections. Parental permission in research involving children, focusing on "not reasonably available." 2018. Available at: https://nam11.safelinks.protection.outlook.com/?url=https%3A%2F%2Fwww.hhs.gov%2Fohrp%2Fsachrp-committee%2Frecommendations%2Fattachment-d-november-13-2018%2Findes.html&data=04%7C01%7Cm.packiam%40elsevier.com%7Cc8e86e3441824dfc3dc508d97a0b4f77%7C9274ee3f94254109a27f9fb15c10675d%7C0%7C0%7C637675011657758073%7CUnknown%7CTWFpbGZsb3d8eyJWIjoiMC4wLjAwMDAiLCJQIjoiV2luMzIiLCJBTiI6Ik1haWwiLCJXVCI6Mn0%3D%7C3000&sdata=E5nEt2YgpuvQ9k5OtZV1%2Fu5ce1P3%2BkUdybBaVdBGGpw%3D&reserved=0. Accessed September 17, 2021.

26. Weijer C, Miller PB. When are research risks reasonable in relation to anticipated benefits? Nat Med 2004;10(6):570–3.

27. Food and Drug Administration. Guidance for industry: acute bacterial otitis media: developing drugs for treatment. 2012. Available at: https://nam11.safelinks.protection.outlook.com/?url=https%3A%2F%2Fwww.fda.gov%2Fregulatory-information%2Fsearch-fda-guidance-documents%2Fguidance-industry-acute-bacterial-otitis-media-developing-drugs-treatment&data=04%7C01%7Cm.packiam%40elsevier.com%7Cc8e86e3441824dfc3dc508d97a0b4f77%7C9274ee3f94254109a27f9fb15c10675d%7C0%7C0%7C637675011657758073%7CUnknown%7CTWFpbGZsb3d8eyJWIjoiMC4wLjAwMDAiLCJQIjoiV2luMzIiLCJBTiI6Ik1haWwiLCJXVCI6Mn0%3D%7C3000&sdata=xni7K8lz83Svd49Puhl80ga6sS3n2Xl1HaXMK%2Bo%2Bar4%3D&reserved=0. Accessed September 17, 2021.

28. Shah S, Whittle A, Wilfond B, et al. How do institutional review boards apply the federal risk and benefit standards for pediatric research? JAMA 2004;291(4):476–82.
29. Appelbaum PS, Grisso T. Assessing patients' capacities to consent to treatment. N Engl J Med 1988;319(25):1635–8.
30. Moser DJ, Schultz SK, Arndt S, et al. Capacity to provide informed consent for participation in schizophrenia and HIV research. Am J Psychiatry 2002;159(7):1201–7.
31. Jeste DV, Palmer BW, Appelbaum PS, et al. A new brief instrument for assessing decisional capacity for clinical research. Arch Gen Psychiatry 2007;64(8):966–74.
32. Kim SY, Caine ED. Utility and limits of the mini mental state examination in evaluating consent capacity in Alzheimer's disease. Psychiatr Serv 2002;53(10):1322–4.
33. Zimmerman M, Clark HL, Multach MD, et al. Have treatment studies of depression become even less generalizable? a review of the inclusion and exclusion criteria used in placebo-controlled antidepressant efficacy trials published during the past 20 years. Mayo Clin Proc 2015;90(9):1180–6.
34. Wong JJ, Jones N, Timko C, et al. Exclusion criteria and generalizability in bipolar disorder treatment trials. Contemp Clin Trials Commun 2018;9:130–4.
35. Hoertel N, Lopez S, Wang S, et al. Generalizability of pharmacological and psychotherapy clinical trial results for borderline personality disorder to community samples. Personal Disord 2015;6(1):81–7.
36. Susukida R, Crum RM, Ebnesajjad C, et al. Generalizability of findings from randomized controlled trials: application to the National Institute of Drug Abuse Clinical Trials Network. Addiction 2017;112(7):1210–9.
37. American Psychiatric Association. Position statement on research with involuntary psychiatric patients. 2018. Available at: https://nam11.safelinks.protection.outlook.com/?url=https%3A%2F%2Fwww.psychiatry.org%2FFile%2520Library%2FAbout-APA%2FOrganization-Documents-Policies%2FPolicies%2FPosition-2018-Research-with-Involuntary-Psychiatric-Patients.pdf&data=04%7C01%7Cm.packiam%40elsevier.com%7Cc8e86e3441824dfc3dc508d97a0b4f77%7C9274ee3f94254109a27f9fb15c10675d%7C0%7C0%7C637675011657758073%7CUnknown%7CTWFpbGZsb3d8eyJWIjoiMC4wLjAwMDAiLCJQIjoiV2luMzIiLCJBTiI6Ik1haWwiLCJXVCI6Mn0%3D%7C3000&sdata=s%2BpfGuL3iERjX%2FMixhw%2F7jvJ8l6dslJ%2BBYs46cFB%2FU%2BE%3D&reserved=0. Accessed September 17, 2021.
38. Review of two mental health patients who died by suicide. Madison, Wisconsin: William S. Middleton Memorial Veterans Hospital; 2018. Available at: https://www.va.gov/oig/pubs/VAOIG-17-02643-239.pdf. Accessed March 15, 2020.
39. Hoge SK, Lidz CW, Eisenberg M, et al. Perceptions of coercion in the admission of voluntary and involuntary psychiatric patients. Int J Law Psychiatry 1997;20(2):167–81.
40. Washington HA. Medical apartheid: the dark history of the medical experimentation on black Americans from colonial times to the present. New York, NY: Random House Digital, Inc; 2006.
41. Bates BR, Harris TM. The Tuskegee Study of Untreated Syphilis and public perceptions of biomedical research: a focus group study. J Natl Med Assoc 2004;96(8):1051–64.
42. Gara MA, Minsky S, Silverstein SM, et al. A naturalistic study of racial disparities in diagnoses at an outpatient behavioral health clinic. Psychiatr Serv 2019;70(2):130–4.
43. Gara MA, Vega WA, Arndt S, et al. Influence of patient race and ethnicity on clinical assessment in patients with affective disorders. Arch Gen Psychiatry 2012;69(6):593–600.

44. Geller SE, Koch AR, Roesch P, et al. The more things change, the more they stay the same: a study to evaluate compliance with inclusion and assessment of women and minorities in randomized controlled trials. Acad Med 2018;93(4): 630–5.
45. McCaskill-Stevens W, McKinney MM, Whitman CG, et al. Increasing minority participation in cancer clinical trials: the minority-based community clinical oncology program experience. J Clin Oncol 2005;23(22):5247–54.
46. Cross-Disorder Group of the Psychiatric Genomics Consortium, Electronic address pmhe, Cross-Disorder Group of the Psychiatric Genomics C. Genomic relationships, novel loci, and pleiotropic mechanisms across eight psychiatric disorders. Cell 2019;179(7):1469–82.e11.

Ethics Oversight in Psychiatry
Data from a Model of Organizational Monitoring

Michelle Hume, MD, PhD[a],*, Kelsey Hobart, MD[b], Laura Briz, MD[c],
Safiah Amara, MD[d], Sean D. Cleary, PhD, MPH[e],
Philip J. Candilis, MD, DFAPA[f,g]

KEYWORDS

- Organizational ethics • Survey • American Psychiatric association
- Ethics complaints • Psychiatrists

KEY POINTS

- This survey of ethics review practices indicates that psychiatrists take ethics review seriously, devoting substantial time and effort to reviewing complaints.
- Complaints against psychiatrists fall into similar categories as previously reported, whereas the number of complaints seems to be declining in recent years.
- Publishing empirical ethics review data and the decision-making behind any subsequent policy changes serve both the transparency and service missions of a professional medical organization.

BACKGROUND

Psychiatric organizations have an important role in setting and monitoring professional and ethical norms. These organizations often represent the public face of the profession, with the ethical behavior of its members influencing the trust and respect earned from both the general public and societal leaders. As part of the social contract and a

[a] Mendota Mental Health Institute, 301 Troy Dr, Madison, WI 53704, USA; [b] Saint Elizabeths Hospital, DC Department of Behavioral Health, 1100 Alabama Avenue Southeast, Washington, DC 20032, USA; [c] Eating Recovery Center/Pathlight, 150 East Huron Street, Chicago, IL 60611, USA; [d] Northeast Ohio Med University, Rootstown, OH 44272, USA; [e] Department of Epidemiology, Milken Institute School of Public Health, The George Washington University, 950 New Hampshire Avenue, Northwest, Suite 500, Washington, DC 20052, USA; [f] Saint Elizabeths Hospital, DC Department of Behavioral Health, 1100 Alabama Avenue Southeast, Washington, DC 20032, USA; [g] George Washington University School of Medicine, Washington, DC, USA
* Corresponding author.
E-mail address: Michelle.Hume@dhs.wisconsin.gov

Psychiatr Clin N Am 44 (2021) 563–570
https://doi.org/10.1016/j.psc.2021.08.004
0193-953X/21/© 2021 Elsevier Inc. All rights reserved.

psych.theclinics.com

moral justification for self-regulation, medical organizations promulgate specific codes of ethics and provide guidance for their members.

The American Psychiatric Association (APA) is the largest and most influential North American psychiatric professional organization, with almost 38,000 members worldwide. Members are guided by the ethical norms and practices described in the APA's Principles of Medical Ethics With Annotations Especially Applicable to Psychiatry (hereafter referred to as the "Principles").[1] The APA's Ethics Committee helps interpret the Principles with the support of its members, consultants, and APA staff. Available resources include educational offerings and commentary, published ethics opinions, responses to specific questions, as well as an ethics primer.[2,3]

The APA delegates the handling of ethics complaints against its members to each of the 72 District Branches (DBs) in 7 regions across the United States and Canada. Each DB adjudicates these complaints according to the Principles as well as peer review policies outlined in its Procedures for Handling Complaints of Unethical Conduct.[4] Most DBs have a standing ethics committee (DBEC) that reviews ethics-related issues. Those DBs without an ethics committee typically use the DB's entire executive committee.

The DBEC reviews the complaint for jurisdiction, then determines whether a recognized ethics violation is alleged. If, after gathering additional information, the DBEC determines the complaint does not allege an ethics violation, the complainant may seek review by the Chair of the APA's Ethics Committee. Depending on the type of complaint and whether it proceeds, the DBEC may decide to offer an Educational Option rather than recommending sanctions. If the responding member does not agree to the Educational Option or one is not offered, the case proceeds to a hearing. The DB then determines whether an ethics violation has occurred and, if so, an appropriate sanction. The responding member may appeal to the APA Ethics Committee.

Formal surveys of ethics complaints were conducted by the APA using data from 1950 to 1983[5] and 2004 to 2007. In the 1985 review, information regarding the number of complaints and number of members affected was obtained from complaints that had been reported to the APA as part of the peer review process. Consequently, complaints that were not sufficiently serious to warrant peer review or were not a violation of the Principles were unlikely to have been counted. In contrast, the survey conducted in 2007 systematically obtained information on all complaints received by DBs, irrespective of how they were resolved. Questions centered on the structure and functioning of the DBECs and the number and typology of complaints and their disposition, including referral to state licensing authorities. DBs were also queried about APA resources that could be helpful in conducting reviews.

This acknowledgment of the importance of transparent monitoring invites the occasional peer or public review of ethics oversight. At its Fall 2019 meeting, the APA Ethics Committee consequently determined that updated data were necessary to inform current practices. Accordingly, committee members with a background in survey design and analysis sought to investigate the number and typology of complaints received by member DBs, the handling of complaints, the relationship between the DB and state licensing authorities, the challenges and resources needed for conducting complaints, and the overall attitude of DBECs regarding ethics review. This analysis presents the results of the survey and outlines how the process may be useful for professional medical organizations adhering to principles of transparency and empirically informed policy.

METHODS

A telephone survey was constructed to address common issues in professional ethics review: the size of committees, the number and type of complaints reviewed, their outcomes, and challenges. The survey was approved by the APA's Institutional Review Board. Open and closed-ended questions were included to allow review of both quantitative and qualitative responses and to permit respondents to identify topics beyond the 17-point questionnaire. Coding of open-ended questions was conducted by agreement of a coding team that piloted the survey among committee members, developed a code book, and reviewed every 5 survey responses for potential adjustments. Any disagreements among coding team members were settled by consultation with the project PIs (MH, PC).

Following an introductory email to DB presidents and DBEC chairs, the survey was administered to responding DBs. Surveys were most frequently conducted with the DB ethics chair, often with the contemporaneous input of the DB executive director. Respondents were advised to answer questions in general terms and not to discuss or disclose information that may identify an individual case or cases. Three to five attempts were made to contact all DBs. Phone contact was attempted if DBs did not respond to email.

In the final analysis, closed-ended questions were tallied and open-ended responses coded. The distribution of responses and their frequencies was examined. Means (with standard deviations) were estimated for continuous variables. To examine differences by group (eg, geographic area, DB size) chi-square tests were used for categorical data and analysis of variance for continuous outcomes.

RESULTS

Overall, 47 of 72 DBs responded, for a response rate of 65%. Within the last 3 years, 23 DBs received 1 to 4 complaints, 18 DBs received 0 complaints, 4 DBs received 5 to 9 complaints, and 2 DBs received 10 or more. The number of complaints was significantly correlated with the size of the DB's membership ($r = 0.63$, $P < .0001$). For every increase of 100 members, there were 5 more complaints received. The size of the branch alone explained 40% of the variance in the number of ethics complaints. There was no significant regional difference in the number of complaints by APA area.

Respondents overwhelmingly believed in the importance of the profession's ethics reviews, rating them 4 or 5 on a 5-point Likert scale (n = 38, 81%). Commonly cited justifications included the demands of an ethical professionalism (n = 23, 49%), the need for a review process (n = 11, 23%), the importance of community trust and protecting patients (n = 7, 15%), and the obligation for psychiatrists to review the behavior of other psychiatrists (n = 5, 11%). Respondents who did not find the reviews important (scoring them 1 or 2 on the 5-point scale, n = 4, 9%) largely cited the availability of state licensing authorities for policing professional behavior.

A total of 95 ethics-related complaints were reported by all respondents in the last 3 years, a rate of 5 complaints per 1000 members. Of these complaints, 22 were eligible for formal peer review, for a rate of 1 complaint per 1000 members. The highest number of peer-reviewed complaints from a single DB was 6. Common reasons for not proceeding with complaints were a lack of evidence, the absence of complainant follow-up, and the complaint being outside of the scope of the DBEC (ie, the complaint was about a nonmember.) Of the 22 complaints that entered formal adjudication, remediation was required in 3 cases. Two psychiatrists received an educational intervention, and one was removed from the APA. Two psychiatrists were reported as has having more than one complaint lodged against them in the study period. DBs generally perceived no change or a decrease in the reporting of complaints over the past 3 years (61% no change, 32% a decrease, 7% an increase). The mean minimum and maximum number of person-hours needed for a complaint were 19 and 32, respectively, with a range of 1 to 100 person-hours depending on the complainant's willingness to follow-up and the nature and complexity of the complaint.

The most frequent type of complaint arose from common practice issues such as disagreements over diagnosis or use of polypharmacy (n = 17, 18%). Boundary violations were the next most prevalent (n = 10, 11%). Smaller numbers related to financial or billing concerns, disagreements over written reports, abandonment, confidentiality, and credentialing (**Table 1**).

DBs valued consultation and contact with APA staff. Eighteen DBs had spoken with APA staff in the last 3 years, and 5 spontaneously commented in positive terms: "wonderful," "knowledgeable," and "helpful." A third of DBs identified APA educational materials as critical to their work (n = 22, 33%). These are the annual ethics refresher courses at APA meetings, mock cases offered during those courses, and online seminars. Respondents specifically identified educational resources posted on the APA Web site, including letter templates for responding to complainants and alerting physicians, and procedural flowsheets. Larger DBs were significantly more likely to report valuing APA educational materials than smaller DBs ($F = 5.47$, $P < .05$). Other DBs reported seeking procedural guidance at times complaints were handled. Approximately 20% (10 of 47) of responding DBs mentioned the availability of the APA Ethics Committee as an important resource in addressing ethical questions. A smaller number described a wish for staff or central office support (**Table 2**).

The challenges outlined by member DBs in conducting ethics reviews are categorized in **Table 3**.

Throughout the survey, numerous responses explored the relationship between DBs and their state's medical boards. Ten DBs (21%) commented on the possibility of redundancy given that both state licensing boards and APA regulate physicians, but another 7 DBs (15%) noted the need for patient protection and for complaints to be heard. Indeed, some respondents raised the possibility that dual review might decrease subsequent complaints. Twelve DBs (26%) reported limited contact with state medical boards. Among DBs with board contact, respondents referred cases to state licensing authorities that were outside the DB's scope, because the complaints related to psychiatrists were either not APA members or were outside the APA's time limit for reporting complaints.

DISCUSSION

This survey of ethics review practices indicates that psychiatrists take ethics review seriously, devoting substantial time and effort to reviewing complaints. The time

Table 1 Ethics complaints by type and number	
Type of Complaint	Number of Complaints of This Type
Practice issue (polypharmacy, diagnostic disputes, and so forth)	17
Boundary violations	10
Jurisdiction	6
Financial/billing	6
Disagreement with a report	4
Abandonment	3
Professionalism, Confidentiality, Credentialing, Goldwater	2 each

Table 2
American Psychiatric Association's ethics resources valued by American Psychiatric Association District Branches

Type of Support	Number of DBs Responding
APA educational materials	22
Procedural guidance	16
Ethics support	10
Staff to assist	6
Central office support	4

commitment reported by DBs is significant and is tied to the nature and seriousness of the complaint. A substantial portion of DBs, greater than 20%, specifically identified the importance of having a professional process by which complainants could be heard. DBs strive for fairness and, even among DBs with fewer members, are committed to fair practices such as the recusal of peers who may have personal or professional ties to responding members.

Respondents appreciate training activities offered through the parent organization. These are mechanisms for review of professional standards and ethics decision-making that standardize review while still allowing the flexibility required by specific cases. Educational offerings such as review courses and mock complaints are specific tools that may resonate across organizations for enriching the connection between the profession's standards and the communities entrusted with ethics review.

That DBs frequently cited educational materials posted on the APA Web site, including letter templates and procedural flowsheets, speaks to the importance of procedural consistency. Survey responses underscore the importance of a readily accessible and streamlined process that allows DBs to focus on the substantive elements of a case. The APA seems to be taking a similar approach to online algorithms used by institutional review boards to determine, for example, whether a study is human subjects research.[6,7]

Survey responses offered consistent support for the review of psychiatrists by other psychiatrists, thus distinguishing APA review from state licensing investigations. Respondents viewed the psychiatric encounter as unique, warranting review by practitioners who were sensitive to the dynamics of the relationship. There was a perception that even complaints that were insufficiently egregious to warrant medical board referral still merited review and required an avenue for the complainant to be heard. Indeed, maintaining a process for frustrated patients may have, for some respondents, reduced the number of times a complaint was filed. Similarly, hospital

Table 3
Challenges of ethics review identified by American Psychiatric Association District Branches

Challenges	Number of DBs Responding
Determining the scope of APA jurisdiction	11
Procedural challenges	8
Logistical challenges	8
Ensuring fairness	5
Recusal	5

systems that have implemented full disclosure policies for unintended outcomes have seen the number of medical malpractice claims, and attorney fees decline significantly.[8–10]

Survey data indicate a significant correlation between the size of the DB and the number of ethics complaints. There was no association between the number of complaints and APA geographic area, although the sample sizes were small. The correlation in number of complaints with size is understandable given the larger universe of psychiatrists in larger DBs. In contrast, prior APA data demonstrated that the percentage of judgements of unethical behavior was nearly 3 times higher in some geographic areas than in others, which seemed unrelated to the number of members.[5] Similarly, a published report of medical board disciplinary actions between 2010 and 2014 found a 4-fold variation in the mean rate of major disciplinary actions by state (2.13–7.93 actions per 1000 physicians)—although not necessarily because of size or geography.[11] Empirical methods such as targeted surveys may distinguish whether membership size truly differs from geography in future analyses and indeed whether these data reflect the range of legitimate ethics options available for interpreting cases or actual regional differences in professional practice.

Because of more numerous complaints, larger DBs reported spending more time on complaints, but it was smaller DBs, likely because of fewer cases, that identified more of an interest in seeking ethics office or committee support. Challenges were predictably related to logistics and procedures. The supportive role of the APA's ethics staff and committee members was consistent across large and small DBs alike, underscoring the dependability, and importance, of central office consultation.

The number of complaints against member psychiatrists seems to be declining in recent years. Between 1950 and 1973,[5] 82 charges of unethical conduct underwent peer review. From 1972 to 1983, the number of peer-reviewed complaints increased to 382 or roughly 40 per year, a rate of 14 per 1000 members. With 65% of current DBs reporting, there have only been 22 peer reviewed complaints in the last 3 years, a rate of 1 complaint per 1000 members.

The finding of substantially fewer complaints is somewhat unexpected given the change in methodology in more recent surveys. As noted previously, both the 2007 survey and the current study asked DBs directly for the number of complaints rather than relying on data reported to APA during the peer review process. As such, in current surveys the authors captured information about complaints that were either not pursued or were handled informally, instead of just those undergoing peer review. Even if all 95 complaints received in the past 3 year were considered, the rate of complaints is still only 5 per 1000 members.

A review of the 2007 survey data confirms a decline in the number of complaints since those data were collected. Present data indicate a lower percentage of DBs with high numbers of complaints than in 2007 (8% vs 4%). Further, the current data demonstrate a higher percentage of DBs with 0 complaints than in 2007 (24% vs 38%) and a lower percentage of DBs with high numbers of complaints. This decline tracks with national statistics on board sanctions against the profession and may reflect the emphasis on ethics education and outreach from the organization and the increased presence of ethics curricula in training programs across the country.

The overall seriousness of complaints also seems to be declining. Of the 82 members charged with unethical conduct between 1950 and 1973, 12 (15%) were found to have acted unethically and 6 were expelled. Between 1972 and 1983, 86 (23%) members were found to have acted unethically and 27 were expelled. The 2007 survey did not ask directly about the number of psychiatrists who were formally sanctioned, but only 6 DBs used this option in the prior 3 years. With only a single expulsion among 22 complaints in the current survey, these data are consistent with the perception of one-third of DB chairs who saw the overall number of complaints decreasing over time. When asked to consider why the number of complaints declined, committee chairs identified procedural changes that emphasized education within the APA and complainants going to state licensing boards rather than to the DBs.

Respondents who underscored the potential overlap between DBECs and state licensing boards raised competing themes. DBECs and state licensing boards may serve different functions, especially because respondents reported little contact with state licensing authorities. There is currently no mechanism by which APA is automatically informed of board complaints. However, complainants do often approach both the board and district branch at the same time. Moreover, when renewing their membership members attest that they will report any action or investigation by a state licensing authority to the APA. Indeed, members who lose their license are no longer eligible for APA membership, so there is a link between licensing and organizational ethics.

The typology of complaints was recognizable from prior surveys, as well as the academic literature. The most common complaints from the 1985 review were patient exploitation and illegal activity, themes that persist in the APA's educational materials. Patient exploitation historically refers to boundary violations, although exploitative fees are included in a more recent edition of the Principles. Although no definition was provided for illegal activity, a survey of 583 disciplined physicians over 30 months in California identified psychiatrists engaging in fraud, tax evasion, selling or writing prescriptions for nontherapeutic drugs, or theft.[12] The current survey echoes the 2007 review, when the most common complaints were boundary issues, incompetent care, and financial or billing issues. Incompetent care has a persistent presence in health care as a whole, with claims for diagnostic errors being especially common in a variety of specialties.[13]

SUMMARY

Policy and oversight that are informed by iterative data collection and review by ethics specialists within an organization may well be a model for maintaining contact with evolving ethics themes in the community. Publishing such data and the decision-making behind any subsequent changes serves both the transparency and service missions of a professional medical organization. Indeed, the view of ethics staff and the organizational Ethics Committee as valued resources suggests a measure of success in achieving educational and collaborative goals among representatives of the profession.

CLINICS CARE POINTS

- Psychiatrists take ethics review seriously and spend considerable time conducting it.
- Psychiatrists appreciate ethics support and training opportunities available through professional organizations.
- Publishing empirical data and the decision-making behind any thematic changes serves both transparency and the service mission of a professional medical organization.

DISCLOSURE

No authors have any commercial or financial conflicts of interest, and there was no dedicated funding source for this article.

REFERENCES

1. American Psychiatric Association. The principles of medical ethics with Annotations especially Applicable to Psychiatry. 2013. Available at. https://www.psychiatry.org/File%20Library/Psychiatrists/Practice/Ethics/principles-medical-ethics.pdf. Accessed December 10, 2020.
2. American Psychiatric Association Ethics Committee. The opinions of the ethics committee on the principles of medical ethics. 2019. Available at. https://www.psychiatry.org/File%20Library/Psychiatrists/Practice/Ethics/Opinions-of-the-Ethics-Committee.pdf. Accessed December 10, 2020.
3. Ethics Primer of the American Psychiatric Association. Washington, D.C.: American Psychiatric Association; 2001.
4. American Psychiatric Association. APA Principles and Procedures for Handling Complaints of Unethical Conduct. Available at: https://www.psychiatry.org/File%20Library/Psychiatrists/Practice/Ethics/complaints-of-unethical-conduct-procedures.pdf.
5. Moore RA. Ethics in the practice of psychiatry: update on the results of enforcement of the code. Am J Psychiatry 1985;142(9):1043–6.
6. University of Wisconsin Health Sciences Educational Review Boards. Guidance on Research vs. quality Improvement and program Evaluation. 2020. Available at: https://kb.wisc.edu/hsirbs/page.php?id=33386. Accessed December 10, 2020.
7. CIRB for the National Cancer Insititute. Algorithm to assess potential Noncompliance. 2017. Available at: https://www.ncicirb.org/institutions/institution-quickguides/managing-study/algorithm-to-assess-noncompliance. Accessed December 10, 2020.
8. Geier P. Emerging med-mal strategy: 'I'm sorry.' Natl Law Journal. July 24, 2006. Available at: https://nam11.safelinks.protection.outlook.com/?url=https%3A%2F%2Fwww.law.com%2Fnationallawjournal&data=04%7C01%7Cm.packiam%40elsevier.com%7Cad6795c2e83f420740d808d979f6265d%7C9274ee3f942 54109a27f9fb15c10675d%7C0%7C0%7C637674921755183189%7CUnknown%7CTWFpbGZsb3d8eyJWIjoiMC4wLjAwMDAiLCJQIjoiV2luMzliLCJBTiI6Ik1haW wiLCJXVCI6Mn0%3D%7C3000&sdata=qcjBcpwu00aQcG0zz4vTvZV4XGA YkjQ5DwZHSeA5orE%3D&reserved=0. Accessed December 10, 2020.
9. O'Reilly KB. Harvard adopts a disclosure and apology policy: for physicians who have erred, "sorry" isn't always an easy thing to say. amednews.com June 12, 2006 November 14, 2020]. Available at: https://amednews.com/article/20060612/profession/306129957/7/. Accessed December 10, 2020.
10. Walling RJ, Ackerman SS. Having to say you're sorry: a more efficient medical malpractice insurance model. Contingencies 2006;18:46–9.
11. Harris JA, Byhoff E. Variations by state in physician disciplinary actions by US medical licensure boards. BMJ Qual Saf 2017;26(3):200–8.
12. Morrison J, Morrison T. Psychiatrists disciplined by a state medical board. Am J Psychiatry 2001;158(3):474–8.
13. Newman-Toker DE, Schaffer AC, Yu-Moe CW, et al. Serious misdiagnosis-related harms in malpractice claims: The "Big Three" - vascular events, infections, and cancers. Diagnosis (Berl) 2019;6(3):227–40.

The Evolution of Forensic Psychiatry Ethics

Philip J. Candilis, MD, DFAPA[a,b,*], Richard Martinez, MD, MH, DLFAPA[c]

KEYWORDS

- Forensic ethics • Forensic psychiatry ethics • Dual agency • Robust professionalism
- Role theory

KEY POINTS

- Ethics at the intersection of Law and Psychiatry are enhanced by models that extend beyond the customary differences in clinical and forensic roles.
- Traditional forensic obligations to Law or Medicine do not take into account the richness of individual and community narratives involved in forensic practice.
- Use of unifying social goals, cultural considerations, and professional identity allows redress of flaws in legal and forensic institutions.

BACKGROUND

When forensic practice was an outgrowth of community psychiatry, it was a simple matter to adhere to common exceptions to general clinical practice, such as civil commitment, guardianship, or Tarasoff warnings. These were special exceptions to the traditional patient-physician relationship that could be justified by obligations to the community. After all, it was the community that privileged physicians, so obligations to society were understood as part of a common social contract for all professions.[1,2] Professionals of all stripes were expected to adhere to licensing rules, practice guidelines, and social expectations. Medical ethics already recognized obligations in several directions: to the patient, to the profession, and to society as a whole.[3]

First among these, however, was unquestionably the duty to the patient. A profession with frankly religious roots, Medicine had evolved as a priestly guild that protected its relationship to patients for centuries dating back to the Ancient Greeks, Rabbi-Physicians, and the Christian Church. The relationship was sacrosanct. However, in forensic psychiatry, traditional patient-physician relationships were the exception rather than the rule.

[a] Saint Elizabeths Hospital, 1100 Alabama Avenue SE, Washington, DC 20032, USA; [b] George Washington University School of Medicine and Health Sciences, Washington, DC, USA; [c] Forensic Psychiatry, CMHI-Ft Logan, 3520 W. Oxford Avenue, Denver, CO 80236, USA
* Corresponding author.
E-mail address: philip.candilis@dc.gov

Psychiatr Clin N Am 44 (2021) 571–578
https://doi.org/10.1016/j.psc.2021.08.001
0193-953X/21/© 2021 Elsevier Inc. All rights reserved.

The difficulty for modern-day forensic psychiatrists was that an entirely different framework applied to clinical thinking when it intersected the legal, correctional, or regulatory systems. The nuanced, team-based, hypothesis testing of the clinic was replaced by the legal system's dichotomous, procedural, dispute resolution.[4] This was a framework with a language and logic all its own. Patients were competent or not, disabled or not, committable or not, sane or not. The Law's definitive judgments were different from the interpretations and inferences drawn by Medicine's clinical reasoning. Advocacy and representation of patient interests were challenged by the traditions and practices of the justice system.

DISCUSSION

The early struggle for forensic psychiatrists centered on the question of whether the physician was guided by the ethical frameworks of Law or Medicine: a classic agency conflict. Whose agent were psychiatrists in the public forum; what role did they play? Did psychiatrists bring their medical profession's ethics to the encounter or adopt the courtroom's? Perhaps there was a hybrid approach that drew on elements of both. In the final analysis, however, if the goals of the Law superseded Medicine when the 2 conflicted, a relationship different than the traditional patient-physician applied for forensic practitioners.

The idea that role determines a professional's action is a powerful one. Commentators frequently suggest that psychiatrists act outside their roles as physicians when they enter the forensic realm.[5–7] Seymour Pollack[8(p18)] was a prominent early proponent of legal primacy for psychiatrists interacting with the law. He observed that,

> Forensic psychiatry in this context is the application of psychiatry to legal issues for legal ends, i.e., for the purposes of legal justice. And it is not primarily concerned with medical or psychiatric treatment of the patient......the psychiatric evaluation of the patient is dominated and controlled by, and directed toward, the specific objectives of the rules of law with which that patient is involved.

Legal goals and purposes were sufficient in this view, and justice was an estimable goal. It may seem quaint in a time of Black Lives Matter and #MeToo, but it is nonetheless a recognizable historical mooring of one's behavior in the obligations of a role. Traced to nineteenth century thinkers like F.H. Bradley,[9(p163)] role theorists defined behavior by its location in certain social constraints and requirements: "We have found ourselves when we have found our station and its duties, our function as an organ in the social organism."

The problem with such classic role requirements is that the role itself provides moral excuses when personal, professional, and community morality conflict. When the legal system, for example, perpetuates inequities of race, gender, and class, mere assumptions of role do little to resolve them. Tame testimony on behalf of a defendant is insufficient to address systemic concerns. The classic Alan Stone[5] "Parable of the Black Sergeant," exemplifies this problem. Stone, a prominent psychiatrist and law professor, famously bade psychiatrists to stay out of the courtroom because they had little to offer a flawed system. He could find little clinical data to support the Black Sergeant when he was accused of theft. There was plenty of evidence of racism and justified anger toward an unjust military system, but no specific exculpatory diagnosis. It would take other writers to move beyond these limitations of role toward a more penetrating professional ethic for forensic psychiatry.

During Pollack's time, it was Bernard Diamond[10(p123)] who took a more clinical stance:

The psychiatrist is no mere technician to be used by the law as the law sees fit, nor [are] the science, art, and definitions of psychiatry and psychology to be re-defined and manipulated by the law as it wishes.

Diamond preferred to be clear that he was the patient's advocate and interested in more therapeutic goals. He was an unabashed supporter of the defense, believing that the power of the state was disproportionate to the resources that could be mustered by the defense. He developed a view of forensic psychiatry that did not accept legal ends blindly. Instead, he considered carefully the potential legal consequences of a case. For him, there was still a place for Medicine's clinical and humanitarian mission when physicians worked with the Law.[11]

Harvard's Thomas Gutheil and colleagues[12] contemporaneously articulated the special differences between clinical and forensic thinking: courts required specific legal answers, whereas clinical analyses incorporated nuances of uncertainty. There was uncertainty in the probabilities and interpretations of science: observations differed among scientists; measurements differed between scales; and analyses differed in their statistical assumptions. However, Gutheil and his group went further. There were institutional tensions as well: civil commitment, for example, raised tensions of values between community safety and patient autonomy, of tensions between facts from actuarial approaches and clinical ones, and of tensions between professions as judges and experts tried to think like each other. Complex social interactions had a context of values and principles that extended beyond dichotomous legal or medical ones.

Other systems theorists like Ciccone and Clements[13,14] found similar room for human values of negotiating and brokering between systems. It was a period that recognized the impossibility of true objectivity. There were always subjective influences on observers, data, and analysis from many quarters, most of which Gutheil and others had already identified. The artificial separation of facts and values (a well-known trap in moral philosophy) gave only simplistic answers to complex social questions like culpability, truth, and justice. Rather, an interdisciplinary relationship between facts and values could relate the medical system to the legal one. A cooperative scheme for science and law was much more satisfying than the assumption of an unattainable ideal like truth.

Such thinking was critical to the introduction of multiple perspectives to the work of Law and Medicine. In 1998, Ezra Griffith[15] pioneered the view that idealizations of truth and justice could not be ethical if flawed systems persisted in their mistreatment of persons of color. Responding to an approach from Paul Appelbaum[7] that prioritized principles of justice and truth-telling for forensic practice, Griffith used the concept of "cultural formulation" to address the inequities between dominant and nondominant groups in the American judicial system. Cultural sensitivity, cross-cultural practice, and narrative were critical for addressing implicit bias and the lack of respect shown to persons of color.

The use of narrative theory was new to forensic ethics, entering at a time that medical ethics itself was beginning to recognize its impact.[16] Narrative, a kind of storytelling truth, exposed some of the sterility of principles in ethics because there were myriad stories describing one's path toward the legal or medical encounter. More nuanced, ambiguous, and indeed, cross-cultural elements of social interactions could be accounted for by narrating the dynamics of social control, disenfranchisement, and inequity.

Of course, ethics was never about principles or narrative alone. Philosopher John Rawls[17] had famously described a "reflective equilibrium" between cases and theory that allowed cases to shape moral judgments as much as principles themselves. This reciprocity enriched theory and clarified how individual cases could be placed in a real-world context. Ethicist John Arras[18(pp71-72)] described this best when he wrote:

> Principles and theories do not emerge full-blown from some empyrean realm of moral truth; rather they always bear the marks of their history, of their coming-to-be through the crucible of stories and cases.

Our own efforts to unify the different approaches to forensic ethics took into account this context of cases and the history of the profession.[19-21] Principles could work at the level of theory, whereas narrative enriched understanding of specific cases. There was a power to uniting personal, professional, and community perspectives into what we termed a robust professionalism.

Acknowledging the subjectivities of perspective when dealing with fraught topics like violence, sex, money, and blame could protect professionals from antiseptic applications of role. Being a technician in a social context that included racism, sexism, and implicit bias was insufficient if the profession were to stand for something. We consequently favored a definition of professionalism from the American Medical Association and its ethicists that acknowledged Griffith's concerns with vulnerable nondominant groups.

Medical professionalism had to be about more than a catalog of characteristics or technical proficiencies. To avoid criticisms of guild protection or self-interest, there was a sturdier moral basis available for any profession's claims of autonomy and self-regulation. Alongside Wynia,[22,23] Griffith, the AMA, and others,[24,25] we underscored the definition of professionalism "as an activity that involves both the distribution of a commodity and the fair allocation of a social good but that is uniquely defined according to moral relationships. Professionalism is a structurally stabilizing, morally protective force in society." Indeed, professionalism must "protect not only vulnerable persons but also vulnerable social values."[22(p1612)]

Here finally was a definition that recognized the moral relationships in a profession's work relationships that were not destructive, but stabilizing and protective. It was not enough to extract information from a forensic evaluee or advocate traditional forensic outcomes, but rather to practice informed consent, provide warnings on the limits of confidentiality, and conduct a cultural formulation.

Vulnerable people were easy enough to identify among those preferentially arrested, incarcerated, and subjected to police violence, but vulnerable values like equality before the bar, representation in policy-making, and advocacy were harder to locate in social institutions that had developed their processes by centuries of self-serving logic. How then could forensic professionals, individually or collectively, advocate for just outcomes without undermining their status, roles, or objectivity?

It may be clear by now that new tools were available for such questions: narrative, cultural formulation, historical context, and perspective could help the contemporary forensic professional. However, there were more as well. An approach in Psychiatry that identified the habits and skills of the ethical practitioner had been in practice for years.[26,27] Experts already knew to educate themselves on the inequities of diagnosis, health care access, the burdens of disease, and the determinants of legal involvement. They could undertake peer review of their cases, consult with colleagues, and reflect on their own blind spots and heuristics. They could be transparent in the reasoning and inferences of their reports and testimony.

Our view that an individual who was in the control of a social institution like a forensic hospital, court, or prison was best described by a story that elevated empathy and compassion,[19(p171)] was advanced by Michael Norko in 2005.[28(p388)] Using religious and secular themes found everywhere from the Bible to Immanuel Kant, Norko pointed out that the Golden Rule, "Do unto others," carried special meaning for a system and profession committed to truth and justice. More than truth-telling or story-telling, compassion allowed professionals "to attend to and engage the humanity of all the subjects of our evaluations."

Norko found that recognizing commonality in all people militated against inequality, incurring obligations of respect for persons that went beyond the usual balancing of one principle against the other. Traditional respect for persons could be outweighed by justice or beneficence, for example, if conditions were right, and despite a foundational narrative of inequity and injustice. Traditional forensic practice without compassion might as well keep forensic experts out of the courtroom as Stone had advised.

Integrating compassion into the identity of the forensic professional supported the evolution from Diamond and his clinical outlook, to Gutheil and Ciccone and their systemic influences, to Griffith and the cultural narrative, and then to the writers on professionalism. Griffith,[29] for example, described how nondominant practitioners brought their own narratives to the work. There were personal, cultural, and community influences on the narratives of forensic experts themselves. After all, they had to function in a system that was insensitive to communities of color.

For us too, professionalism had meant integrating personal, professional, and community values into an identity that retained humanistic and humanitarian ideals.[19] Loyalty to an imperfect system as it currently existed could only coopt the ethics of a profession that honored truth, justice, and fairness. Rather, engaging in compassionate, moral relationships that were sensitive to culture and history could improve the condition of vulnerable people and values. We proposed a concept of professionalism in forensic practice that envisioned the evaluee (or forensic patient) and forensic practitioner situated at the hub of a wheel, with each spoke radiating to the outer rim, a rim that represented the myriad moral relationships in the forensic enterprise.

The forensic professional now incurs an obligation to recognize and consider these relationships and weigh their importance to each connection. Whether in the process of treatment, administrative decisions, or expert opinions and testimony, robust professionalism emphasizes integrity in forensic practice, understood as integration of the whole endeavor. This pattern of moral relationships is foundational to all forensic activities. Mindful reflection and awareness of the many ethics consequences inherent in forensic practice are required. Indeed, the inherent humanity of all patients and evaluees, and the recognition that forensic practice involves the treatment and assessment of vulnerable others, demand compassion and respect.

A new high point for forensic ethics came from the application of human rights theory to the classic tensions between principles and narrative, between precedent and the redress of past inequities. Alec Buchanan[30,31] found new fuel for the evolution of professional ethics in the dignity of persons as the guiding principle of forensic practice. Found in the basic freedoms afforded by liberal democratic principles, from religious and political tolerance to rights of fair trial and fair opportunity, honoring one's inherent worth cut across communities and cultures. It required both cultural sensitivity *and* acknowledgment of unequal treatment.

In a poignant riposte to critics of dignity who saw it as a mere extension of autonomy or respect for persons, Buchanan[30] pointed out that even if slaves were treated with autonomy or respect, their status itself remained an indignity to their inherent value. Thinkers from Aquinas in the thirteenth century to Kant in the eighteenth century had staked out the value of a person's inherent worth.[32]

Human rights grounded in the dignity of persons offered a powerful unifying approach for professional ethics at the intersection of Law and Psychiatry. It still required a concept of professionalism at the practical level to apply the habits and skills of ethical practice, much as principles and narrative functioned at different levels in earlier forensic writings. However, it allowed a broader consideration of the goals and purposes of human interaction even in the most traditional, rule-bound settings. Indeed, Candilis[33] would underscore the usefulness of this construct (human rights plus professionalism) in global mental health, tying risk and other forensic assessments to the cultural and safety requirements of both refugee and host communities in the global refugee crisis.

If the ethics of forensic practice had evolved to consider social justice, systemic racism, and other inequities, the goals and purposes of forensic work had to evolve along with it. Forensic psychiatry had come a long way since the view that forensic consultation was primarily concerned with the ends of the legal system. Martinez and Candilis[34,35] were clear that for forensic psychiatry to remain relevant it must agree on unifying goals that confront the flaws of society. Professional goals and purposes had to evolve to keep up with movements that advanced expanded views of professionalism, and the integration of compassion and dignity into forensic practice.

Alongside traditional forensic goals like providing knowledge of mental illness and competent treatment of persons in forensic settings, Martinez added fundamental practice goals of witnessing, narrating, and decreasing suffering. Indeed, advocating for destigmatization, decriminalization, and nonadversarial approaches in criminal and civil activities enriched outmoded, role-bound thinking in ways that were consistent with the search for overarching social goods. Just as Medicine had identified its core social goods in the 1990s,[36] it was time for the forensic professions to do the same.

SUMMARY

Forensic psychiatry is a relatively young subspecialty. Working at the interface of Medicine and Law, it has required evolution and change to define its ethical coordinates. Developments in the last 50 years have seen it move from a profession acting as a servant to the goals of the Law, to integrating medical and humanistic values. It now defines its own purposes and goals, recognizing that forensic psychiatry interacts with a justice system that is flawed and imperfect. Moving beyond narrow roles and exclusive loyalties, ethical approaches in forensic psychiatry have evolved to allow practitioners nuanced concepts and models for navigating the complex social narratives in the work. Obligations to vulnerable persons and vulnerable values ultimately highlight the proper balance between individual practitioners and institutions that continue to be rooted in structures and traditions that are demonstrably unjust. It is in the unifying ideas of culture, professionalism, dignity, and social goods that forensic commentators have provided guidance to justify their participation at the unique interface of Medicine and the Law.

CLINICS CARE POINTS

Pitfalls of forensic practice
- Ignoring the individual's social, cultural, or institutional disadvantages
- Overlooking misconceptions of the forensic role ("Are you a doctor?")
- Discounting the influence of historical narratives (especially racism, sexism)
- Disregarding established habits and skills of the ethical practitioner (eg, informed consent, confidentiality warnings, education, consultation, cultural formulation)
- Adopting narrow views of the work
- Ignoring obligations to the profession and community

Pearls of forensic practice
- Practice self-awareness, self-reflection
- Monitor personal biases
- Evaluate your own practice trends, case representation
- Prioritize vulnerable persons (eg, inmates, forensic patients)
- Prioritize vulnerable values (eg, access, equity, diversity, representation)
- Consider different models for solving ethics dilemmas (eg, human rights, professionalism)
- Advocate interventions that decrease legal involvement (eg, diversion, housing, outreach)
- Witness and narrate observations of the legal system
- Diminish suffering

DISCLOSURE

The authors have no conflicts to disclose.

REFERENCES

1. Pellegrino ED. Societal duty and moral complicity: the physician's dilemma of divided loyalty. Int J Law Psychiatry 1993;16:371–91.
2. Bonnie R, Monahan J. License as leverage. Int J Ment Health 2004;3(2):134–8.
3. Veatch R. Case studies in medical ethics [Chapter 2]. Cambridge (MA): Harvard University Press; 1977.
4. Candilis PJ, Martinez R. Recent developments in forensic psychiatry ethics. In: Griffith EEH, Norko MA, Buchanan A, et al, editors. Bearing witness to change. Boca Raton (FL): CRC Press; 2017. p. 105–16.
5. Stone AA. The ethics of forensic psychiatry: a view from the ivory tower. In: Stone AA, editor. Law, psychiatry, and morality. Washington, DC: American Psychiatric Press; 1984. p. 15–8.
6. Rosner R. Legal regulation of psychiatry and forensic psychiatry: clarifying categories for physicians. In: Rosner R, editor. Critical issues in American psychiatry and the law, vol. 2. New York: Plenum Press; 1985. p. 19–29.
7. Appelbaum PS. A theory of ethics for forensic psychiatry. J Am Acad Psychiatry Law 1997;25:233–47.
8. Pollack S. The role of psychiatry in the law. Psychiatr Ann 1974;4(8):16–31.
9. Bradley FH. Ethical studies. 2nd edition. Oxford: Oxford University Press; 1988.
10. Diamond BL. The forensic psychiatrist: consultant v. activist in legal doctrine. Bull Am Acad Psychiatry Law 1992;20:119–32.
11. Diamond BL. The simulation of insanity. Journal of Social Therapy 1956;2:158–65.
12. Gutheil TG, Burstajn HJ, Brodsky A, et al. Decision-making in psychiatry and the law. Baltimore (MD): Williams and Wilkins; 1991.
13. Ciccone R, Clements C. The ethical practice of forensic psychiatry. Bull Am Acad Psychiatry Law 1984;112(3):263–77.
14. Ciccone R, Clements C. Commentary: forensic psychiatry and ethics – the voyage continues. J Am Acad Psychiatry Law 2001;29:174–9.
15. Griffith EEH. Ethics in forensic psychiatry: a cultural response to Stone and Appelbaum. J Am Acad Psychiatry Law 1998;26:171–84.
16. Charon R, Montello M, editors. Stories matter: the role of narrative in medical ethics. New York: Routledge; 2002.
17. Rawls J. A theory of justice. Cambridge (MA): Harvard University Press; 1971.
18. Arras J. Nice story, but so what? In H. Nelson, editor. Stories and their limits, narrative approaches to bioethics. New York; Routledge; 1997. p.65-91.

19. Candilis PJ, Martinez R, Dording C. Principles and narrative in forensic psychiatry: toward a robust view of professional role. J Am Acad Psychiatry Law 2001;29: 167–73.
20. Martinez R, Candilis PJ. Commentary: toward a unified theory of personal and professional ethics. J Am Acad Psychiatry Law 2005;33:382–5.
21. Candilis PJ, Martinez R. Commentary: the higher standards of aspirational ethics. J Am Acad Psychiatry Law 2006;34:242–4.
22. Wynia MK, Lathan SR, Kao AC, et al. Medical professionalism in society. N Engl J Med 1999;341:1612–6.
23. Wynia MK, Papadakis MS, Sullivan WM, et al. More than a list of values and desired behaviors: a foundational understanding of medical professionalism. Acad Med 2014;89(5):712–4.
24. Cruess SR, Cruess RL. Professionalism must be taught. BMJ 1997;315:1674–7.
25. Cruess SR, Cruess RL. Understanding medical professionalism: a plea for an inclusive and integrated approach. Med Educ 2008;42(8):755–7.
26. Dyer A. Ethics and psychiatry. Washington, DC: American Psychiatric Press; 1988.
27. Roberts LW, Dyer A. A concise guide to ethics in mental health care. Washington, DC: American Psychiatric Publishing; 2004.
28. Norko MA. Commentary: compassion at the core of forensic ethics. J Am Acad Psychiatry Law 2005;33:386–9.
29. Griffith EEH. Personal narrative and an African-American perspective on medical ethics. J Am Acad Psychiatry Law 2005;33:372–81.
30. Buchanan A. Respect for dignity and forensic psychiatry. Int J Law Psychiatry 2015;41:12–7.
31. Buchanan A. Respect of dignity as an ethical principle in forensic psychiatry. Commentary on 'not just welfare over justice: ethics in forensic consultation'. Legal Criminol Psychol 2014;19:30–2.
32. Rosen M. Dignity: its history and meaning. Cambridge (MA): Harvard University Press; 2012.
33. Candilis P. Arriving at an ethics of global mental health. In: Dyer A, Kohrt B, Candilis P, editors. Global mental health ethics. New York: Springer Publishing Co.; 2021.
34. Martinez R. Professional identity, the goals and purposes of forensic psychiatry, and Dr. Ezra Griffith. J Am Acad Psychiatry Law 2018;46:428–37.
35. Martinez R, Candilis P. Ethics in the time of injustice. J Am Acad Psychiatry Law 2020;48(4):428–30.
36. Hanson MJ, Callahan D, editors. The goals of medicine: the forgotten issues in health care reform. Washington, DC: Georgetown University Press; 1999.

Ethical Considerations in Substance Use Disorders Treatment

Venkata R. Jonnalagadda, MD, DFAPA, DFAACAP[a,b,c,*]

KEYWORDS

- Ethics • Medication-assisted treatment • Opioid • Substance use disorders
- Stigma

KEY POINTS

- Stigma is a critical barrier preventing expansion of substance use disorders treatments.
- Fear that substance use disorders treatments causes addiction needs to be countered with validated research-based training, decisions, and protocols.
- Failure to treat co-occurring physical and mental health diseases while concurrently treating substance use disorders will delay and/or worsen health outcomes.
- There are physicians in active treatment and remission from substance use disorders who can effectively practice medicine.

More than a decade has passed since the last Psychiatric Clinics publication on Ethics in Substance Use Disorders Treatment. Since that time, perspicacity on informed consent, 42 CFR (Code of Federal Regulations) and parity have advanced.[1] There are new challenges in applying the principles of medical ethics to the field of substance use disorders (SUDs) treatment. Issues continue to arise as research investigates the pathology, epidemiology, comorbidity, and regulation of SUDs treatments. It is important for researchers and clinicians to remain rooted in medical ethics as they consider how best to address the public health needs for those affected by SUD and the public policy that seeks to balance the needs of individuals with concerns for public safety. Best ethical practices are especially needed at this time considering the public health crisis of the opioid epidemic in the United States, which has spanned decades and continues to ravage many lives.

Researchers and clinicians have advanced the understanding of SUDs. It is now well-established that SUDs are medical illnesses that require lifelong management

^a Durham VA Healthcare System, Durham, NC, USA; ^b Department of Psychiatric Medicine, East Carolina University School of Medicine, Greenville, NC, USA; ^c Department of Pediatrics, East Carolina University School of Medicine, Greenville, NC, USA
* Greenville VA Healthcare Center, 401 Moye Blvd., Greenville, NC 27834.
E-mail address: Venkata.Jonnalagadda@va.gov

Psychiatr Clin N Am 44 (2021) 579–589
https://doi.org/10.1016/j.psc.2021.08.009
0193-953X/21/© 2021 Elsevier Inc. All rights reserved.
psych.theclinics.com

and treatment much like diabetes, asthma, and heart disease. As new treatment modalities are discovered and refined, concerns have been raised about medication-assisted treatments (MAT). Ethical principles of nonmaleficence and beneficence feature prominently when weighing potential risks with evidence-based research data showing positive outcomes from MAT.

In addition, SUDs have a high comorbidity with other medical and mental health conditions. Comprehensive assessment and treatment of coexisting disorders is needed to address the interacting effects of comorbidities, symptoms of which may serve as triggers for relapse. It is increasingly important for health care providers to work with other professionals and stakeholders in a multidisciplinary/interdisciplinary approach to address relevant health and social determinants.

The 4 principles of medical ethics found in **Table 1** are especially relevant in guiding policy and practices regarding health care professionals with diagnoses of SUDs. Some of the prominent ethical issues in SUDs include access to treatment, reducing stigma to encourage entering treatment, consideration of how some treatments may affect professional competence, and recommendations for further study of MAT and Physician Health Programs for medical professionals with SUDs.

Positive strides have been made in public outreach and understanding of SUDs, recovery advocacy, and refining diagnostic criteria. The Patient Protection and Affordable Care Act, passed in 2010, no longer labels SUDs as preexisting conditions, thereby compelling insurance companies to pay for drug and alcohol treatments, including rehabilitation. Six years later, in 2016, both the Comprehensive Addiction and Recovery Act and the 21st Century Cures Act were signed into law. The first focused on prevention, treatment recovery, criminal justice reform, and overdose rescue. The second promoted more protections for health information, while advancing tele-mental health services, advancing research and development, increasing mental health and SUD treatment access, and creating prescription drug monitoring platforms.

During this same decade, the American Psychiatric Association published the *Diagnostic and Statistical Manual of Mental Disorders* (Fifth Edition) (DSM V) in 2013.[2] DSM

Table 1
Ethical principles and dilemmas related to substance use disorder treatments using the example of opioid use disorder

Principle	Dilemma
Justice • Parity of treatment	Individuals of any background, ethnicity, age, gender, and socioeconomic status can become addicted. However, minors, women, and minority are less likely to receive MAT for a diagnosis of opioid use disorder
Nonmaleficence • Do no harm	One gold-standard treatment of opioid use disorder is buprenorphine. Buprenorphine treatment carries the risk of causing psychological or physical dependence when not paired with behavioral therapies to achieve remission
Beneficence • With good intent	MAT has increased abstinence rates and decreased overdose for those suffering from opioid use disorder. There is a risk of comorbid mental and physical disorders being overlooked by providers, which greatly reduces remission success rates
Autonomy • Freedom of choice	Physicians impaired by opioid use disorder are currently limited in treatment options available to others if they wish to practice medicine. Stringent treatment guidelines for active licensure or to regain licensure discourage MAT best practice standards

IV divided addictions into abuse and dependence, whereas the current DSM 5 combines these into the singular "Use Disorder." For example, Alcohol Abuse and Alcohol Dependence are now Alcohol Use Disorder. Sets of criteria identify a specific Use Disorder (eg, Alcohol Use Disorder, Opioid Use Disorder, Cannabis Use Disorder, etc.). The criterion of legal problems was removed, and the criterion of cravings was added. Each disorder is differentiated by severity: mild, moderate, or severe. These changes in nomenclature reduced diagnostic ambiguity and simultaneously eliminated negatively charged terms identifying individuals suffering from the collective diseases of SUDs, such as abuse, abuser, addict, alcoholic, and others, as well as the stigma of legal involvement/consequences. The movement to finally accept SUDs as scientifically evidenced illnesses and not the result of the consequence of personal choices is slowly changing stigma. This critical shift is furthermore creating opportunities for earlier treatment, supporting efforts, and providing resources to aid lifelong recovery treatment plans for those living with the disease (**Table 2**).

ADDICTION: A LIFELONG ILLNESS

Early recognition of addiction as an illness by physicians came during the eighteenth century. Dr Benjamin Rush, a Founding Father and signatory of the Declaration of Independence, was among the first to connect the concept of addiction to illness. Many decades later, Dr Mangnus Huss published *Alcoholismus Chronicus* (1849) outlining the physical disease of alcohol use disorder. Finally, after much study from 1980 to 1991, the American Medical Association established policies definitively identifying the diseases of addiction.

Recovery, in the context of mental health and SUDs, is a concept spanning the domains from clinical recovery to personal recovery. In the clinical meaning, recovery from a disease event signifies improvement with minimal symptoms. Personal recovery, however, is a much broader construct: it is an individual's lifelong journey of managing a chronic illness while continuously working on a healthy lifestyle and meaningful life, also known as "in remission" from chronic disease. The creation of Alcoholics Anonymous (AA) in 1935 by Bill Wilson and Bob Smith is a globally successful recovery model with the longest experiential demonstration. Similar organizations have emerged for other substances: Narcotics Anonymous, Nicotine Anonymous, Pills Anonymous (for recovery from prescription pill addictions) to name a few. These approaches are available for those seeking support in their struggle with the disease of addiction and generally follow similar meeting platforms, polices, and online presence as AA.

Table 2
Substance use disorders: changes in nomenclature and terminology to reflect a more accurate representation of an accepted chronic disease and reduce stigma

Past	Current
Abuse and dependence	Use disorder
Alcoholic; drug addict	Individual with an alcohol use disorder; substance use disorder
Dirty or popped positive	Positive drug screen
Clean	Abstinent
Reformed addict	Someone in long term recovery; In remission
Opioid replacement; methadone maintenance	Medication-assisted treatment; medications for substance use disorder treatment

The anonymity of these programs is considered essential in providing for the safety of those struggling with SUDs as they work toward sobriety and maintaining remission. Anonymity is a tradition that also protects these programs from public perception that any one individual represents the program itself. These programs also encourage the principle of attraction over promotion, meaning that AA and similar 12-step meetings do not advertise or seek out new recruits. Meetings are open to anyone with a desire to stop using alcohol, whereas additional meetings are available for those who are interested in supporting a member or want to learn more about the programs. These program traditions are important in protecting those seeking treatment from stigma and provide a safe place to listen and share with others. Individuals who do speak publicly about their lived experience with SUDs can bring greater awareness in the fight against stigmas and misinformation held by society at large, but in doing so, they often risk being perceived and treated negatively by others.

The Substance Abuse and Mental Health Services Administration was created in 1992; it has overseen the release of information, and the funding of research and services for SUDs. Even with this advance, the stigma surrounding SUDs has remained significant and continues to be a barrier to treatment and achieving recovery. A 2014 study on public opinion as it relates to SUDs versus mental illnesses found statistically significant discriminatory thought against individuals diagnosed with SUDs.[3] These biases were compelling regarding personal life choices, choices in the workplace, and across society at large, highlighting the prevalence and implications of stigma. For example, persons surveyed were largely unwilling to have an individual diagnosed with a SUD marry into their family or work closely with them in a professional setting.[3] Furthermore, to date, antistigma strategies have found limited success focusing on the individual and community to change false beliefs and build awareness that SUDs are diseases. Plans of action to support antistigma strategies on a bigger global scale have largely been unsuccessful and have not generated lasting awareness.[4] As a matter of ethics and justice, efforts must continue to eliminate stigma and its deleterious effects of creating both barriers to treatment and outright discrimination. The core message requires continuous education in all settings, aimed to broaden the understanding that SUDs are illnesses on par with other chronic conditions such as heart diseases and respiratory diseases. Social change is essential to achieve parity of treatment to help ensure individuals with SUDs receive the same level of care for their illness of addiction as they would for any other chronic disease.[5]

Although the evidence is clear that SUDs can be diagnosed in persons of all ages, genders, and socioeconomic backgrounds, there are still disparities in access to and funding for treatments. Respect for persons in accordance with the principle of autonomy, obligations of advancing health (beneficence), responsibilities to avoid harm (nonmaleficence), and considerations of fair allocation of treatment resources (justice) all support the need to advance accessible and effective treatment of all persons with SUDs. Unfortunately, substantial work must be done to achieve this goal. For example, one of the first SUD pediatric studies from 2001 to 2014 found that only 1 in 4 commercially insured youth with a diagnosis of opioid use disorder received pharmacotherapy, and disparities based on sex, age, and race/ethnicity were evidenced.[6] This study highlights 2 critical issues constraining successful chronic disease management and remissions of SUDs: the disparity in access to treatment and delayed or missed opportunities to initiate treatment. Both issues have harmed individual patients and societal efforts to mitigate the opioid epidemic.[7]

Current solutions aimed at fighting addiction stigma and misinformation have taken multiple forms in recognition of the ethical imperative of advancing access to and treatment of SUDs. For example, these measures have included mandating continuing medical education (CME) licensure requirements for physicians and advanced practice clinicians (physician assistants and nurse practitioners) on safe opioid prescribing practices.[7] Key learning objectives of these educational modules include development of assessment skills, avoiding overprescribing and polypharmacy, and appreciating the risks of abruptly discontinuing medications without safe tapering processes. Additional efforts to promote prevention, treatment, and recovery include increasing awareness through outreach programs to schools, community organizations, government officials, and public service announcements shared with media outlets.[7]

To increase the number of individuals with access to SUD treatment in accordance with the current standard of care, awareness efforts are also extending beyond psychiatry into other medical and mental health disciplines. The inclusion of other professionals in the treatment of individuals with SUDs can help make a meaningful and lasting impact on patients: for example, studies have shown that the expansion of the MAT waiver and the early implementation of treatments have resulted in longer periods of remission and fewer deaths by opioid overdose.[8]

Persons with SUDs may also experience stigma from members of the medical community. Ethical responsibilities of physicians to advance the care of patients and to prevent harm also extend to advancing the public health. However, regarding stigma, there may be a hesitancy on the part of physicians and other professionals to treat patients with SUDs at least in part due to the presumptive long, difficult, and uncertain course of the chronic disease. However, research has shown that relapse rates for SUDs for individuals in treatment are at 40% to 60%, comparable with relapse rates for other common chronic conditions such as cardiac and respiratory illnesses. That being said, there are no quick fixes or definitive cures for SUDs at this time, and it remains true that there is a moderate to high probability of relapse for individuals with SUDs who are in treatment.[7] Relapse can lead to negative life events including job loss, damage to personal relationships, failure to maintain financial obligations, risk of incarceration, and death from overdose. Repeated relapses can be draining for patients as well as providers and concerned spouses, friends, and family members.[7]

Long-term recovery goes beyond initial detoxification, reduction in use, and managing cravings. It is the eventual development of an individual's chronic disease transformation, which includes both physiologic and psychological adjustments in the patient's thought and behavior patterns. Treatment can help individuals develop effective coping skills, move away from negative influences, and change their responses to biological and environmental triggers. These comprehensive changes create lasting, fundamental improvements in an individual's relationships, attitudes, and routines such that lifelong recovery is possible. Against this backdrop, relapses are considered both part of the disease and the treatment process. In order for sustained recovery to be achieved, clinical commitment and mutual trust of the treatment team and the patient is required. Attunement to ethical considerations of respect, treatment, care, harm reduction, and justice can advance and help sustain this critical therapeutic alliance in the setting of treatment setbacks.

CREATING ADDICTIONS, TREATING ADDICTIONS

The opioid epidemic itself raises central ethical concerns about the conduct of pharmaceutical companies and the healing professions. Specifically, as the availability of high-potency opioids and opioid analogues became more widespread and profitable, in the early 2000s, accrediting bodies and federal agencies mandated health care professionals to implement pain management standards often referred to as the "fifth vital sign."[9] The subsequent increase in prescription opioid pain medications began, followed by overdoses and deaths. Although this account is an abridged narrative of a larger set of systemic factors and patterns in health care beyond the scope of this article, the take-home point is that patients who were given large doses of opioid medications became physically dependent over time on these medications as evidenced by the fact that most individuals entering treatment after the year 2010 for opioid use disorder have reported their first use was from a painkiller prescribed by a medical professional.[9] The contribution of prescribing practices to the surging opioid epidemic further reinforces the ethical responsibility of the medical profession to reduce harm to individuals affected by providing treatment and advocacy.

Although public health concerns about opiates are not new, the current opioid epidemic is a true crisis because drug overdose deaths nearly tripled between 1999 and 2014.[10] Between 1999 and 2018, it is estimated that 750,000 Americans died of drug overdoses.[10] Educational mandates, treatment funding, and prescription monitoring programs aided the drop of overdose death rates from 2017 to 2018: according to the Centers for Disease Control and Prevention data, death rates from heroin use decreased by 4% and prescription opioid overdose death rates decreased by 13.5% during that time[10] Continuing this momentum and sustaining reductions in opiate deaths is an ongoing challenge. An early 2019 Harvard-based investigation predicted an increase in overdoses moving forward as those struggling with opioid use disorder seek illicit fentanyl and heroin as alternatives away from MAT programs.[11] In addition, the global coronavirus disease 2019 pandemic was associated with an increase in opiate overdoses and death, with every state in the United States reporting an increase in opiate-related overdoses and other problems during the pandemic.[12] With the pandemic and the intensified and long overdue focus on disparities in health and health care, it is an ethical imperative that persons with SUDs have access to care and are not neglected in accordance with justice considerations.

While measures to manage the opiate epidemic are underway, it is important to contextualize the current public health crisis in the historical context of prior efforts to address opiate use.[13] For example, the opioid epidemic started long before the end of the twentieth century with historical reports describing the treatment of pain using opioids during the Civil War (1861–1865) as well as depicting soldiers struggling with morphine addiction. By 1914, concerns about the overuse of opioids led to the Harrison Narcotics Act, which limited the use of opioids to by prescription only. This cycle of events is forebodingly similar to current policy responses: the desire to mitigate suffering created demand and addiction, with acts of beneficence, unwittingly, seeding an epidemic. In efforts to solve the crisis, restrictions were put in place. With continued demand and increased regulation, alternative illicit pathways emerge to secondary markets offering a dangerous reprieve and often deadly options; in today's opiate epidemic these dangers include the illegal sale of lethal heroin, fentanyl, and diverted prescription opioids.

The examples described previously show the sharp pendulum swings between permissive (and even encouraged) prescribing and the subsequent consequences. Research advances in addiction medicine and information sharing have created immediately applicable partial solutions. Increased education opportunities and opioid-prescribing CME requirements for medical licensure promote knowledge and safe prescribing practices.[14] Prescription drug monitoring programs[15] are dashboards offering accessible prescription data that can be used by prescribers and pharmacists to prevent overprescribing and uninformed prescribing and reduce prescription diversion. Having a patient's current prescription history in real time provides physicians better information to make safer prescribing decisions, and therefore safer treatment determinations.

With new safeguards, supports, the educational availability, and ease of obtaining a MAT waiver, patients should have increased access to opioid use disorder treatments. However, as a 2018 perspectives article in the *New England Journal of Medicine* points out, the waiver and its associated trainings have not increased the needed access for patients to the gold-standard option of MAT.[16] Myths such as buprenorphine is not a solution but a "replacement addiction," or the idea that abstinence is the safe solution to opioid use disorder have caused misplaced fears, precipitated overdoses on illicit alternatives, and delayed positive health outcomes.[16] MAT is not prescription treatment alone but a combination of medication treatment and behavioral therapies. The reality of successful MAT is the creation of a safe way for patients to work on addiction behaviors and triggering cycles in the context of controlled dosage management in combination with structured healthy lifestyle changes to reduce the substantial morbidity and mortality of opiate use disorders. According to the National Center for Health Statistics, from February 2018 to 2019, an estimated 69,000 people died of SUDs, and 7 of 10 were due to opioid overdose specifically.[17] For the year ending in January 2021, however, overdose deaths were up by more than 30%.[18] MAT remains an important component of treatment and one measure to reverse overdose trends. Now more than ever efforts to advance treatment and reduce mortality from SUDs are critical.

ADDRESSING CO-OCCURRING DISORDERS

Advances in multispecialty approaches to health care and interdisciplinary team-based models of care including physical and mental health integration and attention to socioeconomic determinants have shown benefits in prevention, positive health outcomes, and lowering costs by reducing hospitalizations (**Fig. 1**). For persons with co-occurring SUDs and mental health and medical comorbidities, the ethical aims of patient autonomy, beneficence, nonmaleficence, and justice may be best met with a collaborative approach including mental health, primary care, and community-engaged collaboration to navigate and decide among the different providers' and patient's priorities to achieve results born of shared decision making. For example, a patient who has alcohol use disorder, posttraumatic stress disorder, hepatitis, cardiomegaly, and anemia presents with medical complexity that alone requires patient engagement with treatment and multiprovider input and management of diagnostic and therapeutic treatment plans. When braided together with an interdisciplinary team model of adding community engagement to address contributing factors such as homelessness, courts, isolation, poverty, and literacy, the treatment plan can offer healthful solutions for the patient and not just disease control and symptom reduction.

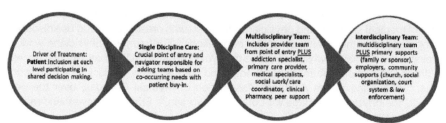

Fig. 1. Comprehensive treatment pathway for substance use disorders (1) impacts stigma, (2) addresses co-occurring illness, and (3) sustains remission with patient-driven, shared decision making.

Broad team-based treatment approaches are critical now more than ever with estimates of as high as 50% of patients seeking treatment of SUDs also carrying a co-occurring psychiatric disorder. Mental illness can make patients more vulnerable to self-medicating and at risk to develop an SUD, and conversely, SUDs can trigger and/or exacerbate symptoms of other mental illnesses. Even more, both SUDs and co-occurring mental illness may be precipitated and exacerbated by the susceptibilities of stress, trauma, and genetic predispositions. According to the National Institute on Drug Abuse, anxiety disorders such as generalized anxiety disorder, panic disorder, and posttraumatic stress disorder are also high-risk diseases linked to SUDs.[19] The intermix of an SUD, a physical disorder, and a mental health disorder exhibits the greatest risk of nonmedical prescription opioid use,[20] thereby underscoring an ethical imperative to effectively address all 3 elements in concert with social determinants to provide just and effective treatment of persons with SUDs as for any other illness.

The time is now as, for the first time in history, an opportunity for sustained success in addiction treatment exists with a comprehensive interdisciplinary treatment approach using MAT. To fully accomplish this clinical and ethical goal, 4 crucial components are required:

1. Prescribers committed to the Integrated Recovery Model trained in the MAT paradigm with waivers, and supported by active psychosocial interventions.
2. Early identification and concurrent treatment of both physical and mental health comorbidities.
3. Patient and support network education and consent regarding evolving paradigms and interventions in SUD recovery.
4. Community stakeholder education and engagement to accept and invest in services and resources for patients in long-term recovery.

This paradigm is not a quick resolution. The disease of addiction is a complex labyrinth to navigate and has potential growing impact: according to the 2018 National Survey on Drug Use and Health 3 of 5 people aged 12 years or older used substances (tobacco, alcohol, illicit drugs) in the month before they were surveyed.[21] With prevalent substance use in the US population, attention to avoiding development of SUDs and treating those that have emerged will require methodical, monitorable prevention and treatment protocols to address SUDs and reduce overdose fatalities. Without investment in these resources, ongoing misunderstanding, failure to treat the whole patient, and ongoing stigma will continue to perpetuate human suffering due to SUDs.

SUBSTANCE USE DISORDERS IN PHYSICIANS

SUDs do not discriminate, and physicians are no exception. Alcohol is identified as the predominant drug of choice of medical students, residents, and physicians, followed closely by prescription medications.[22] In fact, a 2014 study found that greater percentages of medical students and physicians struggled with prescription drug use disorders compared with other members of the population.[22] Furthermore, physicians work in stressful environments, which increases their vulnerability to SUDs; have greater access to drugs and higher probability of burnout; and are less likely to disclose health problems.[23] According to the American Association of Medical Colleges, over the next decade, the physician shortage will continue to worsen.[24] Efforts to prevent and reduce SUDs in physicians are therefore important to the workforce and the public health. These efforts are also important to promote the safe practice of medicine by physicians in upholding public safety and health, and supporting and assisting colleagues with SUDs is part of professional collegiality and self-regulation.

Like other individuals with SUDs, physicians are not immune to the effects of stigma. Multiple factors contributing to stigma include licensure standards with disparate questions about mental health and physical health, fear of liability, concern about loss of licensure long term, and alienation by colleagues.[25] Attention to the effective prevention and treatment of SUDs is critical within the profession across stages of training and of illness. For example, educating and supporting medical students and residents in practicing self-care and remaining vigilant against burnout is a credible prevention model. Early interventions may encourage reluctant health care professionals to come forward for treatment sooner, before problems escalate. For physicians currently in remission from SUDs, who have chosen to access gold-standard treatments, the fear of forever losing their right to practice medicine should not be a penalty for succeeding in chronic illness remission, and medical licensing boards and professional organizations have responsibilities to continue to advance the standard of care for physicians to maintain safe practice.

Specifically, at this time, a central debate with ethical implications for physicians and their ability to practice revolves around the safety of continued practice with MAT given its efficacy as part of long-term sustained recovery. In balancing between safety considerations and physician well-being, more study is needed to understand the cognitive and functional effects of MAT in physicians because this critical area of enquiry presently has limited study data.[26] For physicians with SUDs, principles of beneficence, nonmaleficence, and autonomy must be balanced with the critical responsibility of the profession and licensing agencies to public safety and well-being. In that respect, although what the parameters are for a physician on MAT to practice medicine are yet to be delineated, it is critical to recognize that withholding effective treatments from physicians due to unsubstantiated concerns is problematic and counters professional ethics by potentially withholding safe and effective treatment and simultaneously increasing the risk of professional defeat, or worse overdose and death. At the same time, the protection of the public cannot be sacrificed based on a lack of evidence of harm to meet the desire of a physician with an SUD to resume practice. Ongoing study is needed to inform policy.

SUMMARY

As the push to advance the treatment of SUDs continues and access improves, ethical challenges will continue. "Progress not perfection," is a phrase common in a foundational publication of AA, *Big Book*. This phrase is the discourse of recovery and, so too, the ethics of SUD treatment. As its predecessor in the prior ethics volume of *Psychiatric Clinics*, this article prominently featured the tensions between clinical, ethical, and legal policy approaches to SUDs and the challenges in advancing ethical care. Although psychiatry now recognizes that SUDs are chronic illnesses resulting from many factors, including genetic vulnerabilities, health disparities, clinical exposure, and limited socioeconomic resources, the stigma associated with SUDs continues to create barriers to treatment. As an ethical matter of justice, efforts must continue to both prevent and treat SUDs and their associated morbidity and mortality. Special concern is warranted to evaluate considerations of fairness in availability and access of treatment, inequality in resource distribution, and ongoing challenges in balancing individual rights with the best interest and health of society. The measure of progress will be counted by the number of people living with SUDs who are accepted, treated, and saved and the number who are no longer lost to overdose and medical complications.

CLINICS CARE POINTS

- Justice through antistigma education is needed for patients, health care providers and society at large. The misperception that SUDs are not diseases, and those suffering from them are immoral and dishonest, has created terrible inequities in health care access and treatment to those suffering.

- There is a misapplication of nonmaleficence in choosing not to treat individuals with gold-standard treatments due to apprehensions that SUD treatments create addictions. This misinformation needs to be countered with validated research-based training, decisions, and protocols.

- As health care providers practice beneficence by treating SUDs the failure to concurrently treat co-occurring physical and mental illnesses will delay and/or worsen health outcomes.

- More study is needed to ensure the autonomy of health care providers with SUDs to choose MATs such as buprenorphine, if they can do so safely without harm in the practice of patient care.

DISCLOSURE

The author has nothing to disclose.

REFERENCES

1. Geppert CMA, Bogenschutz MP. Ethics in substance use disorder treatment. Psychiatr Clin 2019;32-2:283–97.
2. American Psychiatric Association. Diagnostic and statistical manual of mental disorders. 5th ed. 2013.
3. Barry CL, McGinty EE, et al. Stigma, discrimination, treatment effectiveness, and policy: public views about drug addiction and mental illness. Psychiatr Serv 2014;65:1269–72.
4. Committee on the Science of Changing Behavioral Health Social Norms; Board on Behavioral, Cognitive, and Sensory Sciences. Division of behavioral and social sciences and education; National academies of sciences, engineering, and medicine. Ending discrimination against people with mental and substance use disorders: the evidence for stigma change. Washington (DC): National Academies Press (US); 2016.
5. Saitz R, Larson MJ, Labelle C, et al. The case for chronic disease management for addiction. J Addict Med 2008;2(2):55–65.
6. Hadland SE, Wharam JF, et al. Trends in receipt of buprenorphine and naltrexone for opioid use disorder among adolescents. JAMA Pediatr 2017;171(8):747–55.
7. Surgeon general's report on alcohol, drugs, and health: early intervention, treatment, and management of substance Use disorders. 2016. Available at: https://addiction.surgeongeneral.gov/executive-summary/report/early-intervention-treatment-and-management-substance-use-disorders.
8. Substance Abuse and Mental Health Services Administration. Medication Assisted Treatment. 2020. Available at: https://www.samhsa.gov/medication-assisted-treatment.
9. Baker DW. The Joint commission's pain standards: origins and evolution. Oakbrook Terrace (IL): The Joint Commission; 2017. Available at. https://www.jointcommission.org/-/media/tjc/documents/resources/pain-management/pain_std_history_web_version_05122017pdf.pdf?db=web&hash=E7D12A5C3BE9DF031F3D8FE0D8509580.

10. Rudd RA, Seth P. Increases in durg and opioid-involved overdose deaths – United States, 2010-2015. MMWR Morb Mortal Wkly Rep 2016;65:1445–52.

11. CDC Press Release. New data show significant changes in drug overdose deaths. Available at: https://www.cdc.gov/media/releases/2020/p0318-data-show-changes-overdose-deaths.html.

12. American Medical Association. Issue brief: nation's drug-related overdose and death epidemic continues to worsen. Available at: https://www.ama-assn.org/system/files/issue-brief-increases-in-opioid-related-overdose.pdf.   Accessed August 15, 2021.

13. Qiushi C, Larochelle R. Prevention of prescription opioid misuse and projected overdose deaths in the United States. JAMA Netw Open 2019;2(2).

14. North Carolina Medical Board. Prescribing CME requirement. 2020. Available at: https://www.ncmedboard.org/landing-page/controlled-substances-cme-requirement.

15. Center for Disease Control and Prevention. What states need to know about prescription drug monitoring programs. 2017. Available at: https://www.cdc.gov/drugoverdose/pdmp/states.html.

16. Wakeman S, Barnett M. Perspective: primary care and the opioid-overdose crisis — Buprenorphine myths and realities. N Engl J Med 2018;379:1–4.

17. Ahmad FB, Rossen LM, Sutton P. Provisional drug overdose death counts. National Center for Health Statistics. 2020. Available at: https://www.cdc.gov/nchs/nvss/vsrr/drug-overdose-data.htm#citation.

18. Centers for Disease Control. 12 Month-ending provisional number of drug overdose deaths, as of 8/1/2021. Available at. https://www.cdc.gov/nchs/nvss/vsrr/drug-overdose-data.htm. Accessed August 15, 2021.

19. NIDA. Common Comorbidities with Substance Use Disorders. National Institute on Drug Abuse website. https://www.drugabuse.gov/publications/research-reports/common-comorbidities-substance-use-disorders. Accessed April 26, 2020.

20. Katz C, El-Gabalawy R. Risk factors for incident nonmedical prescription opioid use and abuse and dependence: results from a longitudinal nationally representative sample. Drug Alcohol Depend 2013;132(1–2):107–13.

21. Substance Abuse and Mental Health Services Administration. (2019). Key substance use and mental health indicators in the United States: results from the 2018 National Survey on drug Use and health (HHS Publication No. PEP19-5068, NSDUH Series H-54).

22. Berge KH, Seppala MD, Schipper AM. Chemical dependency and the physician. Mayo Clin Proc 2009;84(7):625–31.

23. Gold KJ, Andrew LB. "I would never want to have a mental health diagnosis on my record": A survey of female physicians on mental health diagnosis, treatment, and reporting. Gen Hosp Psychiatry 2016;43:51–7.

24. Heiser S. New findings confirm predictions on physician shortages. AAMC Press Release 2019. Available at: https://www.aamc.org/news-insights/press-releases/new-findings-confirm-predictions-physician-shortage.

25. Dumitrascu DI, Mannes PZ. Substance use among physicians and medical students. Med Student Res J 2014;3:27–35.

26. Wollman SC, Hauson AO. Neuropsychological functioning in opioid use disorder: A research synthesis and meta-analysis. Am J Drug Alcohol Abuse 2019;45:11–25.

Ethical Issues in Consultation-Liaison Psychiatry

Marta D. Herschkopf, MD, MSt

KEYWORDS

- Ethics • Consultation-liaison psychiatry • Decisional capacity • Transplant
- Reproductive psychiatry

KEY POINTS

- Psychiatric consults are often called to help address ethical issues; the boundary of the psychiatrist's role in these situations is a topic of debate.
- Mental illness is associated with decreased life expectancy for a variety of reasons; C-L psychiatrists can help facilitate care for this vulnerable population.
- Decision-making capacity is a clinical/ethical determination that is decision specific and may change over time.
- Psychosocial evaluations for transplant and other surgical procedures serve many purposes, including safeguarding informed consent as well as a gatekeeping function in the allocation of scarce resources.
- Treating mental illness in a pregnant patient generally serves both her and the fetus.

INTRODUCTION

Consultation-liaison (C-L) psychiatry has been variably defined and understood. Fundamentally, it is the area of psychiatry that specializes in the care of persons with both medical and psychiatric illnesses, with an understanding that these processes can reinforce and complicate one another. The distinction between the concepts of "medical" and "mental/psychiatric" illness remains an area of controversy within the field, and within psychiatry generally, because it toggles between biomedical and psychological explanatory frameworks in our understanding of disease and mental functioning. Two decades ago, anthropologist Tanya Luhrmann[1] delineated how the legacy of mind-body or mind-brain dualism continues to be played out in American psychiatric education as a tension between biomedical and psychodynamic models. This tension continues, and for C-L psychiatrists, the distinction contains a

Department of Psychiatry, Beth Israel Deaconess Medical Center, Harvard Medical School, Harvard Medical School Center for Bioethics, 375 Longwood Avenue, Masco Suite 370, Boston, MA 02215, USA
E-mail address: mherschk@bidmc.harvard.edu

Psychiatr Clin N Am 44 (2021) 591–601
https://doi.org/10.1016/j.psc.2021.08.008
0193-953X/21/© 2021 Elsevier Inc. All rights reserved.

further consideration of whether a symptom or illness is something that is meant to be addressed by psychiatry or by other medical specialties.

There are many ways that C-L psychiatry addresses issues at the fulcrum of mind, brain, and body.[2] First, there is an appreciation that symptoms of depression, psychosis, and anxiety can be manifestations of pathologic processes that are not generally considered the purview of psychiatrists. For example, psychosis may be a symptom of delirium or cerebrovascular accident or a side effect of steroid medications, and C-L psychiatrists carefully hone their ability to identify these underlying causes and suggest "medical" ways of addressing a "psychiatric" problem. Second, there are a variety of somatoform disorders in which psychopathology presents with "medical" symptoms of pain or neurologic impairment; ironically, the treatment of such disorders often involves "medical" interventions of physical therapy and primary care visits alongside psychotherapy. Third, there are times that the psychological burden of a medical illness may result in a person developing psychiatric symptoms; for example, a patient who becomes depressed after a diagnosis of advanced cancer. And finally, although there is growing research into both the biological and psychosocial underpinnings of "psychiatric" illnesses such as schizophrenia and major depressive disorder, the scientific community has not yet identified reliable biomarkers to aid in psychiatric diagnosis.[3]

Psychiatrists play a myriad of roles within society, and C-L psychiatrists situated at the intersection of medicine, psychiatry, and systems of care are often called upon to wear many different hats. C-L psychiatrists are beholden to a variety of stakeholders, including patients, families, medical staff, and society at large. Recognizing and balancing conflicting ethical responsibilities to these parties is part of the daily work of the C-L psychiatrist.

A separate but important role of C-L psychiatrists generally may be to advocate on behalf of patients with concomitant medical and psychiatric illness, or at the very least, to help facilitate their care.[4] Severe mental illness is associated with a significant mortality gap; patients with schizophrenia, for example, tend to die an average of 13 to 15 years earlier than the general population.[5] There are a variety of reasons for this difference including patient-level factors, such as higher rates of behaviors associated with chronic illness (eg, substance use, poor diet) and difficulty adhering to medical care/visits. However, there are also provider-level factors, including discriminatory beliefs about the ability of patients with severe mental illness to care for themselves and/or participate in their own health care decisions, as well as the phenomenon of "diagnostic overshadowing," when physical symptoms are more likely to be attributed to mental illness rather than medical illness.[6] Systems-level factors include lack of access to care and the siloing of psychiatric care from other forms of medical care delivery.[6]

This article focuses on 3 common areas in which the work of C-L psychiatrists is all but inextricably intertwined with ethical principles and analysis: decisional capacity assessment, transplant evaluations, and evaluations in the context of reproductive medicine. First, determination of decisional capacity is generally taught to all physicians in medical ethics courses, and often in clinical training as well, as part of respecting patients' autonomy and engaging in the process of informed consent. In practice, however, it is generally C-L psychiatrists who are asked to evaluate decisional capacity if there are doubts about a patient's ability to make an informed decision or the decision is high stakes in terms of medical or perceived liability risk.[7] The role of psychosocial evaluations in allocating transplants and other resources is another area in which C-L psychiatrists are faced with important ethical considerations around principles of justice and beneficence in the course of clinical care. Finally, in the setting of reproductive psychiatry, C-L psychiatrists must not only care for the identified patient, but there is the additional stakeholder of an unborn child, raising ethical issues of beneficence, nonmaleficence, and the potential for conflicting obligations.

History of Consultation-Liaison Psychiatry

In Western biomedical culture, the idea that "psychiatric" illnesses might have "medical" causes has its roots in the nineteenth century. In the early twentieth century, American psychiatrists began to argue that rather than being regulated to asylums, they had a role to play within the general medical hospital, both to start treating mental illness proactively within a medical framework and to help treat patients whose mental symptoms were interfering with medical/surgical treatment.[8,9] Psychiatrists were also seen as important advocates to combat the stigma of mental illness, and there was an early appreciation of the ways that psychiatrists might help avoid unnecessary medical/surgical intervention if a patient's symptoms were seen to represent mental rather than physical illness. The field grew in the 1930s to the 1940s, while at the same time starting to be influenced by psychoanalysis; this was the genesis for another name for the specialty, "psychosomatic medicine," which emphasized the interplay of biological and psychological factors in the genesis of disease (both "psychiatric" and "medical").[8,9]

In the second half of the twentieth century, C-L programs expanded in the United States and had a growing emphasis not only on "consultation" activities of diagnosing and treating mental illness but also on a psychologically and psychoanalytically based "liaison" role of working to educate nonpsychiatric staff about the biopsychosocial model, including discussions of staff transference and countertransference reactions. This liaison role waned in later years as a result of both funding issues and a more general move within psychiatry away from psychoanalytic theory.[8,9] Nonetheless, C-L psychiatrists have retained and developed important liaison roles in assisting medical and surgical colleagues in navigating the many relationships and systems inherent in health care.

In addition, although C-L psychiatry has its origins in hospital-based practice, it grew in the latter half of the twentieth century to include community-based psychiatrists integrating with primary care physicians and other specialty clinics. Outpatient-oriented sub-sub-specialty interests in, for example, human immunodeficiency virus psychiatry, reproductive psychiatry, psycho-oncology, and transplant psychiatry became subsumed within the C-L framework. In the early twenty-first century, there remains a great deal of optimism and enthusiasm of the role that C-L psychiatry might play within a variety of systems.[8,9]

Ethics and Consultation-Liaison Psychiatry

A 2006 survey of C-L psychiatrists found that nearly all respondents saw themselves as being involved in clinical work with significant bioethical aspects, although few had formal training in bioethics.[10] Many scholars have pointed out that psychiatry consultations are often ethics consultations in disguise. Four decades ago, for example, a 1982 *New England Journal of Medicine* commentary suggested that one reason for the prominence of ethics in psychiatric consultations is that "Psychiatrists are seen by their colleagues as having added training in dealing with conflict, including moral conflict, as being more reflective, and as having more time to assess the situation."[11] Consulting teams may also be looking for ways to offload the emotional and logistical labor of ethically fraught situation, consciously or unconsciously. This tendency is seen in other psychiatry- and ethics-adjacent fields, such as palliative care[12] and social work,[13] who are also often consulted to help address a variety of ethical issues.

The role of a consultation psychiatrist in a case with psychiatric and ethical components is a subject of controversy. Lederberg[14] warns of the danger of psychiatrists acting like amateur ethicists, and of ethicists acting like amateur psychiatrists, but goes on to argue that psychiatrists specialize in understanding the nonrational, psychosocial components of ethical reasoning. Hayes[15] argues that the C-L psychiatrist does have a role to play in moral arbitration, particularly when ethics consultation may not be available, and provides schemas to help psychiatrists educate themselves about ethical inquiry. Kontos and colleagues[16] suggest that the role of a consultation psychiatrist may be to identify an underlying ethical issue, but not necessarily to resolve it.

Autonomy and Decisional Capacity

Many ethical challenges within C-L psychiatry arise in the context of evaluations of decisional capacity. Decisional capacity is a threshold consideration within the ethico-legal concept of informed consent, based on the principle of autonomy, that a person has the right to determine what happens to their body;[17] this reflects a shift in the medical community in the latter half of the twentieth century, moving away from a more parentalistic, beneficence-based ethical approach in which the physician assumed the responsibility to decide what was in the patient's best interests.[18]

Decisional capacity is itself an ethical construct, and there is some controversy about whether psychiatrists or ethics consultants are better suited to making determinations about decisional capacity.[19] Although there are some ethics consultants who directly opine on decisional capacity, it is also common to defer to psychiatric consultants on this topic, particularly when an ethics consult service sees itself as identifying a variety of ethically acceptable options, rather than making clinical (or ethical) recommendations.

The assessment of decisional capacity is classically based on the evaluation of 4 criteria. These are the ability to (1) communicate a choice, (2) understand the relevant information, (3) appreciate the situation and its consequences, (4) reason about treatment options.[20,21] There is a general appreciation that the stringency of the standard applied occurs on a "sliding scale" based on the relative risk of an intervention (or nonintervention), with more risky or seemingly "irrational" decisions requiring a robust demonstration of capacity by the patient.[18] It is important to emphasize that this determination of how strict a standard to apply is fundamentally an ethical question, and one that has not and does not get as much attention in the psychiatric literature as do other, more technical aspects of capacity consultation.

C-L psychiatrists have at times belabored the distinction between a clinical determination of incapacity, made by a doctor, and a legal determination of incompetence, made by a court. Capacity is a fluid clinical-ethical construct, with a patient potentially having capacity for some decisions and not others, whereas the related legal/ethical concept of competence is generally applied more comprehensively and broadly, although legal standards do recognize spheres of competence. Capacity (or competence) is described in the bioethics literature as a threshold criterion for informed consent; put another way, a patient who is incompetent will, by definition, lack the ability to provide informed consent for any medical decision.[17] That said, these terms are often used interchangeably in practice, with many requests for consultation to determine "competence." Given that to legally act on a determination of incapacity a patient generally must be legally declared incompetent, the distinction between the 2 terms is often less relevant to the consult itself.[21] That said, medical teams often need to be reminded that a psychiatric determination of decisional incapacity/incompetence does not justify coercive measures alone, but must be upheld through the appropriate legal channels and use of substituted judgment.[22] In practice, decisions about capacity and determinations of incapacity do not rise to the level of formal legal or judicial intervention given the growing and now widespread use of advance directives such as health care proxies, in particular following the passage of the 1990 federal legislation.[22]

Decisional capacity determinations are often ethically fraught. Clinical uncertainty can have dramatic consequences because a psychiatrist must distill a complex evaluation into a yes/no dichotomy regarding who can make decisions about a patient's care. A determination of "lacks capacity" may be used to justify coercive treatment measures for a patient, whereas a determination of "demonstrates capacity" may be used to justify neglect. Indeed, moving from a parentalism-oriented framework to an autonomy-oriented one may overemphasize a simplistic, and seemingly unlimited, conception of autonomy that ultimately does not respect the patient's personhood.[23,24]

Related to this point, the framework of a decisional capacity consult that weighs autonomy against other competing principles has come to be overutilized as a model of resolving unrelated ethical issues.[16] A 2017 retrospective review of one institution's decisional capacity consults over a year-long period found that 56.8% of them were "unwarranted," that is, "not at all about the cognitive aspects of a patient's [decision-making capacity]."[7] Some examples of such "unwarranted consults" are cases in which patients obviously lack decision-making capacity, or when a team questions decision-making capacity based on a psychiatric diagnosis alone rather than observed impairment in actual decision making. The investigators also provide examples of decisional capacity consults apparently driven by moral distress or legal concerns.[7]

Psychiatry consultants can often be helpful in unfocused or "unwarranted" decisional capacity consultations, even if, in the end, no direct assessment of capacity occurs. Clinically in these situations, C-L psychiatrists can help identify specific factors that may be compromising the ability to make and/or communicate decisions and suggest ways to address/reverse the causes. From a liaison perspective, they can provide education about the determination of decisional capacity and legal steps that follow it (while also directing teams to legal or social work resources). A psychiatric diagnosis/formulation can also be helpful in guiding care more broadly. Psychiatry consultants may also be able to help teams identify the ethical problem underlying the consultation request and direct them to more appropriate resources for addressing it (such as an ethics consult).[16,25] That said, access to ethics consultation may not be available in every clinical setting or in the time frame required for time-sensitive decisions. In such cases, individual psychiatric consultants may choose to educate themselves further to acquire the knowledge and skills to engage in the ethical analysis and/ or discussions that arise related to capacity and other consults, or may prefer to limit their role.[25]

Finally, although beyond the scope of this review, an emerging area at the intersection of capacity assessment and ethics is the determination of decisional capacity to request physician-assisted death and/or euthanasia in states/countries in which it has been legalized,[26] and more generally, the role of psychiatric disorders in the determination of capacity and/or as a grounds for requesting medical assistance in dying.

Justice, Transplants, and Gatekeepers

A second area of C-L practice with prominent ethical overlap and implications is the psychosocial evaluation of patients before organ/tissue transplants. Of note, psychiatric assessment is increasingly a precursor for other medical and surgical interventions, such as bariatric surgery and medical and surgical gender affirmation. Such evaluations not only address the ability to engage in informed consent but also place C-L psychiatrists front and center in bioethical debates regarding the allocation of scarce resources and as de facto gatekeepers.

The purposes of presurgical evaluations are severalfold. First, they are meant to ensure that patients are able to engage in informed consent about a high-risk procedure that requires a commitment to subsequent medical follow-up and treatment. For example, transplants generally include lifelong immunosuppression, which carries substantial risks in itself.[27] For vascularized composite allotransplantation (commonly referred to as quality-of-life transplants, including face, hand, penile, or uterine transplants), it is important for patients to have realistic expectations of outcomes and subsequent functioning before consenting to what is not a life-saving but may be a life-enhancing surgical intervention.[28] For example, some hand transplant recipients have subsequently requested that the hand be removed, because they found that the functional benefits were less than what they had anticipated, and the rehabilitation and transplant care burdens greater than expected.[29]

Second, from the perspective of beneficence/nonmaleficence, pretransplant evaluations also address psychiatric symptoms that might be exacerbated by the treatment and/or interfere with the ability to maintain adherence to postsurgical recommendations. This determination is relevant not only to individual outcome but also to maximize the utility of organs allocated for transplant and prevent waste. A comprehensive psychosocial evaluation will identify these factors as well as (hopefully) treatment plans to mitigate the risks they present.[27]

However, these evaluations serve another role, namely, a gatekeeping function. In other words, certain patients may be excluded as transplant candidates if there is evidence that they will not be able to adhere to posttransplant care, due to concomitant psychiatric illness (such as addiction) or a lack of social supports and/or resources. It is, therefore, important for C-L psychiatrists to understand that a discussion of this gatekeeper function as well as the limits of confidentiality of the assessment are part of informed consent to participate in the psychosocial assessment itself.[27] Although published guidelines on organ allocation generally list socioeconomic status and contribution of the patient to their own medical condition as inappropriate criteria for allocation decisions,[30] they also list substance dependence and psychiatric illness associated with medical nonadherence as valid contraindications to transplant listing, because they are predictive of limited likely benefit from the procedure.[30,31] Some critics have argued that the implementation of psychosocial criteria can be systematically discriminatory against those with mental disabilities, because such patients often lack robust psychosocial supports and may struggle with medical adherence.[32]

These considerations bring to the fore varying conceptions of justice in the allocation of scarce resources. A utilitarian concept of justice emphasizes trying to maximize good outcomes, often aligning with the ethical principle of beneficence, and also leaving open the possibility that allocating an organ to the person who would take care of the organ best and extend its useful life may not be beneficent for an individual excluded from receiving an organ due to factors arguing that the individual would not be a good steward of the limited resource. An egalitarian concept of justice, based on the work of John Rawls as applied to health and health care by Norman Daniels, emphasizes social justice considerations of allocating interventions in ways that maximize equal access to social benefits. An implication of this approach is to give precedence to those who are the worst off in terms of health or social opportunities, particularly if their poor health is due to unequal distribution of the social determinants of health.[33,34]

In making allocation decisions, transplant committees must balance different ethical considerations for a variety of stakeholders (patients, donors, health care workers, society at large) as well as different conceptions of justice. C-L psychiatrists play de facto roles as both gatekeepers and advocates in this process. Transplant programs may also promote the ability of persons with mental illness to safely and effectively undergo transplantation by devoting resources to facilitate access to mental health treatment of candidates both before and after surgery.

Psychosocial evaluation is being increasingly required for surgical procedures that do not involve allocation of a scarce resource. These procedures include bariatric surgery, left ventricular assist device placement, some cosmetic surgeries and pain mitigation procedures, gender affirmation surgery, and some assistive reproductive technology. The goals of these evaluations include informed consent as well as a consideration of how psychiatric comorbidities may affect the risk-benefit profile of the procedure, including whether the procedure is likely to be effective. Bariatric surgery, for example, may not be offered to someone suffering from certain eating disorders (such as active bulimia nervosa) or substance abuse, because these behaviors can be particularly dangerous in the postsurgical period.[35] That said, critics have raised concerns about the gatekeeping function of such evaluations given that there is a lack of evidence about their accuracy in predicting surgical outcomes.[36]

It should be noted that psychosocial evaluations are also typically required for living organ donors. These evaluations also focus on informed consent, but with more of an emphasis on ascertaining that the donation is voluntary rather than coerced.[37]

Reproductive Psychiatry and Conflicting Duties

Many ethical dilemmas encountered in C-L psychiatry are related to balancing ethical responsibilities to different stakeholders. A patient's needs may conflict with the needs of their family or caregivers, for example, Although traditional medical ethics generally prioritizes the needs and claims of the patient first, there are, nonetheless, times that other duties and considerations may override patient claims. If a patient is threatening hospital staff, for example, the rights of staff to a safe work environment may supersede the patient's right to exercise self-determination because of the potential harm to others, in this case hospital personnel.

One area in which competing responsibilities may be particularly complex is in the reproductive context. Reproductive psychiatry is a growing subspecialty at the intersection of women's mental health and C-L psychiatry; it focuses on mental health and the treatment of psychiatric disorders in women during the reproductive years, often balancing the care and treatment needs of a pregnant woman or mother who may be experiencing symptom exacerbations due to hormonal shifts and/or other stressors against potential exposures of a fetus or nursing infant to medication.

The moral status of and duties toward an unborn fetus are age-old and remain an ongoing debate in biomedical ethics,[38] yet it is worth noting that there is a legacy in reproductive health care of at times privileging the perceived needs of a fetus over those of the mother. Pregnant women have been criminally prosecuted for illicit drug use as well as medical decisions that could potentially harm the fetus (with disproportional prosecution of poor black women).[39] Similarly, mentally competent pregnant women have been coerced into treatment for the sake of their fetuses, and the American College of Obstetricians and Gynecologists (ACOG) has issued a consensus statement against this practice, specifically noting that "Pregnancy is not an exception to the principle that a decisionally capable patient has the right to refuse treatment."[40] Recent guidance in the literature similarly suggests that there should always be a presumption of decisional capacity for pregnant patients, and that pregnant patients with compromised decisional capacity due to active major mental illness still be involved in medical decision making to the extent possible.[41]

There has also been increased awareness recently that the interests of the mother and fetus generally coincide rather than diverge.[40] Decisions about the use of psychotropic medications during pregnancy previously focused on a dichotomy of treating the mother's illness versus exposing the fetus to risk, whereas research has shown that untreated mental illness is itself an "exposure" for the fetus. Untreated maternal depression, for example, is associated with low birth weight, preterm birth, higher cortisol levels in neonates, increased neonatal intensive care unit admissions, and other postnatal complications.[42] Many traditional studies compared pregnancies exposed to psychotropic drugs against healthy controls without mental illness, which limits their applicability.[43] Thus, modern guidelines prioritize keeping the pregnant woman psychiatrically well while reducing the exposures to the fetus as possible.[42,43] There are also times that a pregnant woman's decisional capacity is compromised, and she is making decisions that jeopardize her own safety as well as that of her fetus. In these situations, coercive treatment may be justified as an option of last resort, with careful consideration of the woman's interests as well as those of the fetus.[41]

SUMMARY

C-L psychiatry focuses on the care of persons with both medical and psychiatric illnesses, with an understanding that these processes can reinforce and complicate one another. Working at the interface of the medial and mental health system, C-L psychiatrists can be important advocates for patient care and also serve as resources to our other medical colleagues. There are a variety of ethical issues that can arise from working within complex systems, particularly with vulnerable patients. This article focused on 3 main areas as exemplary of common ethical issues encountered by C-L psychiatrists: decisional capacity assessment, psychosocial evaluation and allocation of organ transplants, and reproductive psychiatry.

CLINICS CARE POINTS

- Mental illness is associated with decreased life expectancy for a variety of reasons, including patient-level factors as well as discrimination at the level of medical providers and systems. C-L psychiatrists can help facilitate care for this vulnerable population.

- There is a long history of psychiatric consults being called to help address ethical issues; writers differ regarding the boundaries of the psychiatrist's role in such situations.

- Decision-making capacity is a clinical/ethical determination that is decision specific and may change over time. Competence for informed consent is a global legal/ethical determination used to guide decisions about surrogate decision making. The terms are often used interchangeably in clinical and legal contexts.

- Many requests for decision-making capacity consults may be motivated by ethical concerns; a consultant can help teams identify relevant ethical questions and direct them to more appropriate resources to resolve them. A consultant can also be helpful in such consults by providing a psychiatric formulation and treatment/management recommendations.

- Psychosocial evaluations for transplant and other surgical procedures serve many purposes, including safeguarding informed consent as well as a gatekeeping function in the allocation of scarce resources. Different conceptions of justice support different allocation procedures.

- As per ACOG guidelines, pregnancy is not an exception to the principle that a competent patient has the right to refuse treatment.

- The needs of a pregnant woman and the fetus are generally aligned.
- Recent research suggests that the risks of psychotropic medications to a fetus during pregnancy may have been overstated, because there are also risks from exposure to untreated mental illness.

DISCLOSURE

The author has nothing to disclose.

REFERENCES

1. Luhrmann TM. Of two minds: the growing disorder in American psychiatry. New York: Knopf; 2001.
2. Levenson JL. Preface. In: Levenson JL, editor. The American psychiatric publishing textbook of psychosomatic medicine and consultation-liaison psychiatry. 3rd edition. Washington DC: American Psychiatric Association Publishing; 2019. Available at: https://doi-org.ezp-prod1.hul.harvard.edu/10.1176/appi.books.9781615371990. Accessed August 19, 2021.
3. Lozupone M, La Montagna M, D'Urso F, et al. The role of biomarkers in psychiatry. Adv Exp Med Biol 2019;1118:135–62.
4. Rudolph K, Brendel RW. Advocacy for patients in medical settings. In: Vance MC, Kennedy KG, Wiechers IR, et al, editors. A psychiatrist's guide to advocacy. Washington, D.C.: American Psychiatric Association Publishing; 2020. p. 453–78.
5. Hjorthøj C, Stürup AE, McGrath JJ, et al. Years of potential life lost and life expectancy in schizophrenia: a systematic review and meta-analysis. Lancet Psychiatry 2017;4(4):295–301.
6. Viron MJ, Stern TA. The impact of serious mental illness on health and healthcare. Psychosomatics 2010;51(6):458–65.
7. Pesanti S, Hamm B, Esplin B, et al. Capacity evaluation requests in the medical setting: a retrospective analysis of underlying psychosocial and ethical factors. Psychosomatics 2017;58(5):483–9.
8. Schwab JJ. Consultation-liaison psychiatry: a historical overview. Psychosomatics 1989;30(3):245–54.
9. Ali S, Ernst C, Pacheco M, et al. Consultation-liaison psychiatry: how far have we come? Curr Psychiatry Rep 2006;8:215–22.
10. Bourgeois JA, Cohen MA, Geppert CMA. The role of psychosomatic-medicine psychiatrists in bioethics: a survey study of members of the academy of psychosomatic medicine. Psychosomatics 2006;47(6):520–6.
11. Perl M, Shlep EE. Psychiatric consultation masking moral dilemmas in medicine. N Engl J Med 1982;307:618–21.
12. Carter BA, Wocial LD. Ethics and palliative care: which consultant and when? Am J Hosp Palliat Care 2012;29(2):146–50.
13. Landau R. Ethical dilemmas in general hospitals: social workers' contribution to ethical decision-making. Soc Work Health Care 2001;32:75–92.
14. Lederberg MS. Making a situational diagnosis. Psychiatrists at the interface of psychiatry and ethics in the consultation-liaison setting. Psychosomatics 1997;38(4):327–38.
15. Hayes JR. Consultation-liaison psychiatry and clinical ethics: a model for consultation and teaching. Gen Hosp Psychiatry 1986;8(6):415–8.

16. Kontos N, Freudenreich O, Querques J. Beyond capacity: identifying ethical dilemmas underlying capacity evaluation requests. Psychosomatics 2013;54(2): 103–10.
17. Beauchamp TL, Childress JF. Respect for autonomy. In: Principles of biomedical ethics. 7th edition. New York: Oxford University Press; 2013. p. 101–49.
18. Drane JF. The many faces of competency. Hastings Cent Rep 1985;15(2):17–21.
19. Schneider PL, Bramstedt KA. When psychiatry and bioethics disagree about patient decision making capacity (DMC). J Med Ethics 2006;32(2):90–3.
20. Appelbaum PS, Grisso T. Assessing patients' capacities to consent to treatment. N Engl J Med 1988;319:1635–8.
21. Appelbaum PS. Assessment of patients' competence to consent to treatment. N Engl J Med 2007;357:1834–40.
22. Brendel RW, Schouten R. Legal concerns in psychosomatic medicine. Psychiatr Clin North Am 2007;30(4):663–76.
23. Childress JF. The place of autonomy in bioethics. Hastings Cent Rep 1990; 20(1):12–7.
24. Stirrat GM, Gill R. Autonomy in medical ethics after O'Neill. J Med Ethics 2005;31: 127–30.
25. Wright MT, Roberts LW. A basic decision-making approach to common ethical issues on consultation-liaison psychiatry. Psychiatr Clin North Am 2009;32(2): 315–28.
26. Bourgeois JA, Mariano MT, Wilkins JM, et al. Physician-assisted death psychiatric assessment: a standardized protocol to conform to the California end of life option act. Psychosomatics 2018;59(5):441–51.
27. Olbrisch ME. Ethical issues in psychological evaluation of patients for organ transplant surgery. Rehabil Psychol 1996;41(1):53–71.
28. Kumnig M, Jowsey-Gregoire SG. Key psychological challenges in vascularized composite allotransplantation. World J Transplant 2016;6(1):91–102.
29. Errico M, Metcalfe NH, Platt A. History and ethics of hand transplants. JRSM Short Rep 2012;3(10):74.
30. Clarke OW, Glasson J, Epps CH Jr, et al. Ethical considerations in the allocation of organs and other scarce medical resources among patients. Arch Intern Med 1995;155(1):29–40.
31. Weill D, Benden C, Corris PA, et al. A consensus document for the selection of lung transplant candidates: 2014—an update from the pulmonary transplantation council of the international society for heart and lung transplantation. J Heart Lung Transplant 2015;34(1):1–15.
32. Orentlicher D. Psychosocial assessment of organ transplant candidates and the Americans with disabilities act. Gen Hosp Psychiatry 1996;18:5S–12S.
33. Daniels N. Justice, health, and healthcare. Am J Bioeth 2001;1:2–16.
34. van der Wilt GJ. Cost-effectiveness analysis of health care services, and concepts of distributive justice. Health Care Anal 1994;2:296–306.
35. Snyder AG. Psychological assessment of the patient undergoing bariatric surgery. Ochsner J 2009;9(3):144–8.
36. Rouleau CR, Rash JA, Mothersill KJ. Ethical issues in the psychosocial assessment of bariatric surgery candidates. J Health Psychol 2016;21(7):1457–71.
37. Jowsey SG, Schneekloth TD. Psychosocial factors in living organ donation: clinical and ethical challenges. Transplant Rev. 2008;22(3):192–5.
38. Beauchamp TL, Childress JF. Moral status. In: Principles of biomedical ethics. 7th edition. New York: Oxford University Press; 2013. p. 62–100.

39. Goodwin M. How the criminalization of pregnancy robs women of reproductive autonomy. Hastings Cent Rep 2017;47(6):S19–27.
40. American College of Obstetricians and Gynecologists. Refusal of medically recommended treatment during pregnancy. Committee Opinion No. 664. Obstet Gynecol 2016;127:e175–82.
41. Babbitt KE, Bailey KJ, Coverdale JH, et al. Professionally responsible intrapartum management of patients with major mental disorders. Am J Obstet 2014;210(1): 27–31.
42. American College of Obstetricians and Gynecologists. Use of psychiatric medications during pregnancy and lactation. Practice Bulletin No. 92. Obstet Gynecol 2008;111(4):1001–20.
43. Chisolm MS, Payne JL. Management of psychotropic drugs during pregnancy. Br Med J 2015;351:h5918.

Severe and Enduring Anorexia Nervosa and Futility: A Time for Every Purpose?

Patricia Westmoreland, MD[a,*], Libby Parks, LCSW[b,1],
Kristen Lohse, PsyD[c,1], Philip Mehler, MD[d,1]

KEYWORDS

- Anorexia nervosa • Futility • Harm reduction • Palliative care • Ethics

KEY POINTS

- Individuals with severe and enduring anorexia nervosa require careful consideration of treatment plans that may include harm reduction, palliative care, and/or end-of-life care.
- Ethical and medicolegal issues arise in individuals with severe and enduring anorexia nervosa.
- The treatment of individuals with severe and enduring anorexia nervosa should consider burden on caregivers and expenditure of health care resources.

INTRODUCTION

Anorexia nervosa (AN) can be a treatable and ultimately curable mental illness. Individuals with AN have the ability to recover even after they have been ill for more than 2 decades, suggesting that active treatment, rather than palliative care, should be considered.[1] Although recovery after such a prolonged course of illness is theoretically possible, for the approximately 20% of individuals who have been unremittingly ill with AN for 8 to 12 years despite multiple attempts at treatment, full recovery is deemed unlikely.[2–4] Individuals suffering from severe and enduring AN (SE-AN) are a subgroup of patients whose illness, although chronic, is not necessarily imminently life-threatening. They are often profoundly underweight (body mass index of <13) and may be physically disabled as a consequence of chronic malnutrition. The physical sequelae of a long-standing eating disorder can include osteoporosis (resulting in a lifelong increased risk of fragility fractures), renal failure, bowel dysfunction (eg, gastroparesis, colonic dysfunction owing to longstanding laxative use), and cognitive

[a] Women's Unit, The Medical Center of Aurora and Consultant, ACUTE Center for Eating Disorders at Denver Health, Denver, CO 80204, USA; [b] Clinical Social Work, ACUTE Center for Eating Disorders at Denver Health, Denver, CO 80204, USA; [c] ACUTE Center for Eating Disorders at Denver Health, Denver, CO 80204, USA; [d] ACUTE at Denver Health, Denver, CO 80204, USA
[1] Present address: 723 Delaware Street, Denver CO, 80204.
* Corresponding author. 50 S Steele Street, Suite 460, Denver, CO 80209.
E-mail address: Patricia.westmoreland@gmail.com

Psychiatr Clin N Am 44 (2021) 603–611
https://doi.org/10.1016/j.psc.2021.08.003
0193-953X/21/Published by Elsevier Inc.

Abbreviations	
AN	Anorexia nervosa
SE-AN	Severe and enduring anorexia nervosa

dysfunction. These individuals are often as impaired by their symptoms as those who suffer from other serious chronic mental illnesses, such as schizophrenia or bipolar disorder, and may not be able to work or live alone. In addition, their ongoing needs for assistance with tasks of daily living places a substantial burden on caregivers.

Individuals with SE-AN require the regular attention of a multidisciplinary team to remain alive, despite a less than optimal quality of life.[3-5] Stigmatization is common in individuals with SE-AN. Thin to the point that they attract stares, they may become isolated socially and depressed. Outpatient clinicians may decline to work with them owing to their medical and psychiatric complexities. Those suffering from SE-AN have often experienced multiple treatment failures and are thus reluctant to engage in further treatment designed to return them to a normal body weight with an ongoing plan of sustaining that weight, despite this approach conferring an optimal prognosis.[6,7]

Therefore managing—and caring for—individuals with SE-AN requires careful consideration of their unique needs and goals versus achieving full recovery. It also requires immense empathy and the ability to be realistic about the odds of effecting a cure.[2] The long-term risk of SE-AN and limited effectiveness of treatment in long-term remission and quality of life present an ethical challenge centered on tensions between helping and healing (beneficence), not harming (nonmaleficence), and respecting persons (autonomy). In other words, the severity and chronicity of SE-AN present circumstances that at least in some cases shift the ethical assessment of how to treat the patient away from seeking cure to decreasing (rather than eliminating) medical harm and individual suffering. Three approaches to treating persons with SE-AN that emerge from this analysis are harm reduction, palliative care, and end-of-life and/or hospice care.

Harm reduction is directed toward maintaining a minimal level of function for the individual involved while decreasing the risks of SE-AN. The goal of a harm reduction model calls for some weight restoration until a lower than optimal, but nonetheless safer and more functional, weight than where the patient started is reached, rather than forcing the individual to undergo a full course of treatment with a limited chance of success and the even likelihood of harm given prior ineffective treatment courses for most persons with SE-AN. The emphasis is not to reach an ideal body weight, but to find meaning and purpose in life, even if these individuals remain somewhat frail and require assistance with tasks of daily living. Although the harm reduction model may decrease the risk of imminent death, individuals undergoing care under a harm reduction model nevertheless remain at great risk of morbidity and early mortality if they develop medical problems such as a viral gastroenteritis, pneumonia, or a fracture.[3,4] Patients in harm reduction treatment should also be monitored for depression, hopelessness, and suicidal ideation, because people who are habituated to pain owing to their physical experiences pose a potential risk for high-lethality suicide attempts. Following a harm reduction approach to treatment for SE-AN should an individual need to be hospitalized for physical or psychiatric decline, the goals would remain to restore the amount of weight they have lost and/or achieve a less unsafe weight, normalize laboratory results, and/or provide crisis stabilization.

Palliative care in SE-AN involves managing pain and other problematic and bothersome symptoms, with the goal of optimizing the individual's quality of life. Although the term palliative care (ie, symptomatic relief from pain or physical or mental stress) is not synonymous with hospice care, these terms are frequently conflated.[8] Palliative care does not necessarily mean preparing for the end of life, but instead optimizing care for the individual through the cooperation between palliative specialists and disciplines and thereby decreasing physical and psychic pain.[9] Individuals with SE-AN who undergo palliative care are those for whom any further treatment (be it with the goal of normalizing weight or achieving weight sufficient for harm reduction) is unlikely to resolve or decrease their illness and suffering. A palliative care focus shifts the goals of care from weight restoration and cure to maximizing the individual's quality of life and decreasing their symptom burden.

Although the goal of easing an individual toward the end of his or her life is well-accepted for medical patients, is a topic of considerable debate with regard to psychiatric patients. There is a distinction between allowing an individual to refuse nutrition and hence end his or her life (the concept of futility), and providing the means with which to assist that person in ending his or her life (physician-assisted death) or actually administering the medicine that leads to death (euthanasia). It is critical to appreciate the differences in these approaches, because each treatment recommendation can significantly impact both quality and duration of life. A such, this review specifically addresses concepts of futility, decision-making capacity, and physician-assisted death as they relate to SE-AN. It also outline the ethical and medicolegal issues that arise in individuals with SE-AN.

DISCUSSION
Futility in Anorexia Nervosa

The concept of futility has sparked a contentious debate as it pertains to eating disorders. Opponents of accepting futility quote data indicating that most potentially lethal medical complications of AN are treatable, in contrast with incurable diseases such as metastatic cancer or neurodegenerative diseases.[10] Indeed, the aforementioned study by Eddy and colleagues[1] demonstrated that cure is possible for individuals with AN even after 20 years of illness, thus making it difficult to label AN as incurable.

However, even though the life of a starving individual may be saved (compared with that of someone with incurable cancer), an individual's refusal to eat engenders a challenging legal and ethical situation.[11] Although nasogastric feeding can be used to restore weight in individuals who refuse food, a determined patient can take out their nasogastric tube, unless he or she is chemically or physically restrained. Force feeding in such a manner is controversial, with much of the controversy arising from the World Medical Association's response to forced feedings of hunger strikers.[11] Simply stated, the coercive nature of forced feeding itself erodes individual autonomy, may threaten personal integrity, has the very real potential to harm patients who have already suffered trauma through retraumatization, and can also damage the doctor–patient relationship and thereby challenge and/or erode the success of future treatment. In contrast, respecting a patient's wishes to stop treatment may represent effectively collusion with the symptoms of a devastating illness at a time when there is an intervention available to save an individual's life. Additionally, there may be a question of the individual's decisional capacity to make treatment decisions about refusing interventions based on the neuropsychiatric and psychological effects of malnutrition and even starvation that accompany SE-AN.

The threshold assessment for an individual's ability to make medical decisions of informed consent and/or refusal is decisional capacity, or an individual's ability to understand information regarding his or her condition, reason through the information needed to make a decision regarding his or her care, appreciate the consequences of the decision he or she makes, and communicate his or her choice.[12] The decision maker must both understand the information presented to him or her and the consequences of making (or not making) the decision for a decision to be considered informed and respected by care providers.[11] It is thus questionable whether individuals with severe eating disorders have the capacity to decide that further treatment is futile when the core symptom of their illness centers on cognitive distortion, most commonly the refusal to believe that starvation is life threatening. In other words, poor insight into the nature and gravity of the illness is caused by the eating disorder itself. There is also a threshold in starvation-related states, which also occurs in eating disorders, at which individuals exhibit a decline in cognition because of chemical changes in their brains.[13] This effect was replicated in a Minnesota study when male volunteers starved to well below their ideal body weight developed behaviors around food akin to those seen in individuals whose starved state is a result of an eating disorder.[14]

As stated elsewhere in this article, individuals with eating disorders frequently lack decisional capacity for multiple reasons. Their characteristic difficulties with thought processing and overvalued ideas are but one aspect of the manifestations of SE-AN that present a serious challenge to competence.[15] Cognitive deficits regarding intolerance of uncertainty and short-sightedness regarding the future also contribute to deficits in decision-making.[16] Individuals with severe eating disorders often say they want to live, but then eschew the very treatment (nutrition) that is required to save their lives, defying the requirement of rationality for decision capacity. Restated, a severely ill patient stating that they wish to live, but then rejecting life-saving care, is not compatible with demonstrating the requisite decisional capacity for medical intervention and certainly not to refuse potentially life-saving interventions.

Involuntary treatment, however, is controversial owing to the autonomy of the patient coming into tension with the obligation of health care professionals to save lives.[17] Because cognitive distortions often can resolve with weight gain, it has been suggested that physicians treating individuals with eating disorders may be compelled to provide treatment, even involuntary treatment, to patients with AN in the hope that, when they achieve a healthier body weight, their cognitive distortions resolve and their decision-making is no longer impaired.[8] For individuals who are incompetent to refuse treatment and who meet the criteria for dangerousness to self and/or grave disability, involuntary treatment can be a useful modality in treating life-threatening eating disorders in the immediate time course.[18,19] Individuals who are treated on an involuntary basis are frequently those who are the most severely and chronically ill, and who therefore face the greatest risk of death. However, although their clinical condition meets the ethical criteria and legal burden of proof required for certification for involuntary treatment (ie, they can be certified), this does not necessarily mean these patients should be certified.[20] Patients who have been chronically ill may not ultimately benefit from inpatient treatment that centers on the goal of full weight restoration, and there may well be a point at which this type of treatment (even if mandated) is futile[21] or even harmful, given the risks of trauma and retraumatization, as well as ongoing distress and suffering.

Specifically, although individuals with SE-AN are often deemed incompetent regarding decisional capacity, these same patients are persons who have had a lengthy lived experience of their illness and its effect on their quality of life. They are typically knowledgeable and insightful as to whether and how their quality of life has improved as a result of treatment in the past. Determining the best course of action for an individual with SE-AN means balancing the ethical principles of autonomy (allowing an individual to make a decision on his or her own), beneficence (making a decision for the good of another individual), nonmaleficence (the principle of first do no harm), justice (ensuring that an individual is treated fairly), and duty to protect (when an eating disorder threatens the life of an individual, taking action to keep that individual safe). There is an inherent subjectivity in weighing these ethical principles. Physicians should recognize their own personal biases and invite other stakeholders into the decision-making process (eg, the individual herself or himself, family members, and long-time treatment providers) to avoid explicit or unintended imposition of their own beliefs and preferences in patients' care. In addition, the right decision may vary at different times during treatment, depending on an overall balancing of factors, thus making it important to assess for capacity and the individual's circumstances on an ongoing basis in the context of the individual's life and not just the present circumstances that may provide overwhelming support for time-sensitive intervention in the acute setting.

The following cases illustrate the ethical and legal challenges in treating individuals with SE-AN when they refuse treatment while under medical care. Ultimately, the course of events and determinations resulted in the death of both patients. At the time they refused treatment, both individuals seemed to lack capacity. First, a 24-year-old woman in the United Kingdom who had suffered from AN for at least 7 years, was hospitalized on 11 occasions over 5 years and involuntarily treated with nasogastric feeding and psychotropic medication. At the time of her hospice admission, she was severely underweight and suffering from pressure sores, urinary incontinence, and multiple fractures as a result of SE-AN. She continued to exercise despite knowing the risk that continuing to exercise (in the setting of lumbar spine fractures) could lead to paraplegia. A week after admission to the hospice unit, she developed delirium and died. Members of the Royal College of Psychiatrists special interest group in eating disorders questioned the death as the result of a failure to try a full range of treatment options and also cautioned that, with AN, a desire for death may be associated with depression, and may fluctuate over time and with the course of the illness.[22]

In a second case, a 30-year-old patient with SE-AN, Lopez and colleagues[23] noted that forcing her into involuntary treatment, or waiting for her to voluntarily engage in treatment, were unlikely to cure her eating disorder or afford her a reasonable quality of life. Despite the termination of active care and the initiation of hospice care, the patient was reluctant to discuss end-of-life issues, and insisted both that she would not die and did not want to die. Her health continued to decline, and she died 3 weeks after admission to a hospice care unit. Despite questions about her capacity, her treatment team asked, "Even if she had been declared legally incompetent regarding her ability to make treatment decisions, then what?" They indicated that capacity may not be the final arbiter in deciding whether to initiate end-of-life care. Instead, they explored how to think about care interventions when a patient with SE-AN who has a poor prognosis (eg, seems to be facing a terminal course) and continues to decline physiologically and psychologically, should be given the more humane choice of hospice care versus forcible interventions that had an undoubtedly questionable prognosis.[23] Another case review described patients who had been assessed in terms of decision-making when they elected to pursue end-of-life care and who also chose to succumb to their illness.[24] These patients were older than those described by O'Neil and Lopez and their colleagues, had longer periods of failed treatments, and their refusals of life sustaining care had been consistent over a long period of time.[23,25]

Two legal cases from the United Kingdom argue opposing sides of the futility debate as it pertains to SE-AN. In *Local Authority vs. E*, a patient with SE-AN had previously executed advance directives refusing compulsory feeding.[26] Her parents and physicians argued that she was comparatively well when she executed the directives and asked that her wishes be honored, even if doing so would result in her death. The judge opined that Ms E suffered from similar cognitive distortions at the time of the court hearing as she did when she executed the directives, and that the value of life overrides the presumption that further treatment will fail. The court ordered that Ms E be force fed involuntarily. A critic of the judge's decision suggested that supporting the wishes of the patient and the family may have been better at promoting autonomy and well-being than saving the life of a patient who did not want to engage in further treatment, and whose family supported her decision.[27]

In *NHS Foundation Trust vs. Ms. X*, Ms X, who had suffered from AN for 14 years, opposed being force fed.[28] Although Ms X reportedly lacked capacity, the judge ruled in her favor and opined that forced feeding against her wishes was inhumane and interfered with her autonomy. The judge also noted that, although forced feeding (resulting in weight gain) can be mandated, psychological treatment cannot be forced. However, this line of reasoning failed to take into consideration that weight gain improves cognition and enables patients to engage therapeutically.[6,7]

In *Re. Miss W*, Miss W at age 28 had suffered from SE-AN for 20 years and had 6 prior admissions for inpatient treatment, amounting to a total of 10 years spent in inpatient care, more than one-third of her life.[29] After a subsequent decrease in Miss W's weight, the Health Board raised 2 contrasting proposals for consideration. The first option was for Miss W to be refed under sedation, which involved her being unconscious for 6 months and being tube fed, and the second option was to discharge to her parents' home with a community support program. In adjudicating this case, the Judge opined it was "beyond the power of the court to bring about an improvement in W's circumstances or an extension of her life," and Miss W's discharge to the community was the "least worst option."[29]

In 2016, a court in the United States also ruled that a 29-year-old woman with severe AN had the right to refuse forced feeding. A.G., whose weight was approximately 69 lbs, was involuntarily committed to a psychiatric hospital in New Jersey. Her guardian had previously obtained a court order for surgical placement of a gastrostomy tube to forcibly feed A.G. to save her life. A.G. subsequently experienced refeeding syndrome and heart failure and removed the tube.[30] The guardian then petitioned the court to allow A.G. to enter palliative care. Members of the bioethics committee concluded that A.G. was capable of making her own medical decisions. The state argued that A.G. was not capable of making informed decisions about her treatment. Judge Paul Armstrong pronounced that A.G.'s testimony was "forthright, responsive, knowing, intelligent, voluntary, steadfast and credible" and that she knew death was a possible outcome.[30] The court did not rule on her competency, but adopted a paradigm of cooperative spirit of the patient, parents, treatment team, and ethics committee of the hospital. The result was a uniform voice that reflected an amalgamation of autonomy, beneficence, and nonmaleficence. A.G. subsequently died in February of 2017. A.G.'s case seem to be the first time a US court upheld the right of a patient with AN to refuse tube feeding and other treatment, even when it ultimately led to their death. Because this case ended at a trial level with no official reported opinions or appellate review, the case is limited in its precedential weight with regard to setting a binding legal guidance.[31]

Several months later, the same judge presided over the case of S.A. At 20 years old, S.A. had severe AN since age 13. In 2017, she was admitted to an acute care hospital weighing 60 lbs. Her psychiatrist and medical doctors believed she was delusional, in denial, and did not understand her risk of dying and therefore did not have the capacity to make her own medical decisions. S.A.'s parents petitioned the court to override their daughter's refusal of treatment and to provide involuntary feeding to save her life. S.A. articulated her wishes to return home and manage her own easting disorder and described being in treatment as "torture." The judge opined that SA's parents were acting in her best interest to save her life and that S.A. had neither reached the same stage of organ failure and grave functional debility as A.G., nor had she endured as many years of failed inpatient treatment.[32] He granted the parents guardianship over her medical decisions.

Taken together, these challenging cases and their legal resolutions highlight the complexity of considerations and ethical analysis inherent in making decisions for patients with SE-AN who are both severely ill and in need of treatment while being in opposition to treatment owing to a combination of disease, personal lived experience, and autonomy considerations that call into question the general standards of decisional capacity assessment but also invoke an appeal to fundamental humanity and compassion. Further work is needed to continue to understand the clinical and ethical features of relevance and applicability to persons with SE-AN to advance compassionate and competent medical treatment for them.

Framework for the End of Decision-Making in Eating Disorders

Some psychiatrists and eating disorder professionals oppose palliative and end of life care for patients with SE-AN, citing concern regarding a "slippery slope" argument that would make all patients with SE-AN inherently eligible for support in making choices to end their lives rather than receive aggressive and potentially life-saving care. Proponents of this view note that the illness itself often compromises a patient's ability to make a fully competent decision, and therefore that overriding a patient's wishes may be justified under the doctrines of parentalism and care in an effort to save that patient's life and return him or her to a state where she or he can make an informed and competent decisions. On the other side, there is justifiable reluctance on the part of eating disorder professionals to undertake any treatment that bears little hope of advancing a patient's quality of life, directly opposes the wishes of that patient and family, and extends a life of suffering, even if the patient has diminished capacity. Yet, physicians are also reluctant to give up hope. In the end, this hope should be balanced by a careful assessment of each individual's circumstances so that patients are not forced into an intolerable living situation merely because they are deemed to lack capacity. Even if a patient lacks decision-making capacity, he or she is still likely capable of appraising his or her suffering.[33,34] Futility should therefore be considered on a case-by-case basis when considering a particular treatment intervention, at a particular time, for a particular patient.

A framework proposed in 2015 incorporates these considerations in recommending that decisions regarding further episodes of care for individuals with Se-AN should be made (1) at a time when the patient is competent (ie, ideally between episodes), (2) the individual must know that refusing nutrition will lead to death (3) the individual's decision to die must be based on a realistic assessment of current quality of life, and the low probability that current or future treatment will succeed, and (4) individuals must be consistent in communicating their desires.[35]

SUMMARY

Ethical decisions in treatment for individuals with SE-AN are fraught with ambiguity and complexity and each case must be thoughtfully considered. It is important to realistically assess each individual's capacity for recovery as well as their ability to engage in a harm reduction or palliative care model as opposed to a treatment model aimed at cure. It is important to remain informed of the wishes of the patient, their family, and their treatment team. Additionally, the burden on caregivers and stewardship over the expenditure of health care resources should also be considered when deciding whether traditional treatment (whether voluntary or involuntary), harm reduction, palliative care, or end-of-life care be recommended for a particular individual. End-of-life care is controversial, but it may be of expanding relevance for a small set of patients with AN whose illness is severe and enduring. Using this type of care should only be as a result of an extensive and well-considered decision-making process. In addition, failure to consider end-of-life comfort-focused care as an option for individuals with a chronic and severe psychiatric illness such as SE-AN may perpetuate the stigma of mental illness as separate from physical illness and discredit the pain and suffering endured by these persons.

CLINICS CARE POINTS

- Treatment plans for individuals with severe and enduring eating disorders often include nonconventional care plans such as harm reduction, palliative care, and/or end-of-life care.
- Capacity should be assessed in individuals with SE-AN who are considering end-of*life care, although capacity may not be the ultimate determining factor.
- Quality of life should be assessed in individuals who do not want further treatment.
- Caregiver burnout and stewardship of health care resources should also be taken into account.

REFERENCES

1. Eddy KT, Tabri N, Thomas JJ, et al. Recovery from anorexia nervosa and bulimia nervosa at 22-year follow-up. J Clin Psychiatry 2017;78(2):184–9.
2. Yager J. Managing patients with severe and enduring anorexia nervosa: when is enough enough? J Nerv Ment Dis 2020;208(4):277–82.
3. Robinson P. Severe and enduring eating disorder (SEED). Management of complex presentations of anorexia and bulimia nervosa. Oxford: Wiley-Blackwell Press; 2009.
4. Robinson P. Severe and enduring eating disorders: recognition and management. Adv Psychiatr Treat 2014;20(6):392–401.
5. Hay P, Touyz S. Treatment of patients with severe and enduring eating disorders. Curr Opin Psychiatry 2015;28(6):473–7.
6. Lund BC, Hernandez ER, Yates WR, Mitchell JR. Rate of inpatient weight restoration predicts outcome in anorexia nervosa. Int J Eat Disord 2009;42(4):301–5.
7. Steinhausen H-C, Grigoroiu-Serbanescu M, Boyadjieva S, et al. The relevance of body weight in medium-term to long-term course of adolescent anorexia nervosa. Findings from a multisite study. Int J Eat Disord 2009;42(1):9–25.
8. Geppert CMA. Futility in chronic anorexia nervosa: a concept whose time has not yet come. Am J Bioeth 2015;15(7):34–43.
9. Trachsel M, Wild V, Biller-Andorno N, et al. Compulsory treatment in chronic anorexia nervosa by all means? Searching for a middle ground between a curative and palliative approach. Am J Bioeth 2015;15(7):55–6.
10. Westmoreland P, Krantz MJ, Mehler PS. Medical complications of anorexia nervosa and bulimia nervosa. Am J Med 2016;129(1):30–7.
11. Boyle S. How should the law determine capacity to refuse treatment for anorexia? Int J Law Psychiatry 2019;64:250–9.
12. Appelbaum PS, Grisso T. Assessing patients' capacities to consent to treatment. N Engl J Med 1988;319(25):1635–8.

13. Matusek JA, O'Dougherty Wright M. Ethical dilemmas in treating clients with eating disorders: a review and application of an integrative ethical decision-making model. Eur Eat Disord Rev 2010;18(6):434–52.
14. Keyes A, Brozec J, Henschel A, et al. The biology of human starvation, vol. 1 and 2. Minneapolis, MN: University of Minnesota Press; 1950.
15. Tan J, Stewart A, Fitzpatrick R, Hope T. Competence to make treatment decisions in anorexia nervosa: thinking processes and values. Philos Psychiatr Psychol 2006;13(4):267–82.
16. Adoue C, Jaussent I, Olié E, Beziat S, et al. A further assessment of decision-making in anorexia nervosa. Eur Psychiatry 2015;30(1):121–7.
17. Tury F, Szalai T, Szumska I. Compulsory treatment in eating disorders: control, provocation and the coercion paradox. J Clin Psychol 2019;75(8):1444–54.
18. Westmoreland P, Mehler PS. Caring for patients with severe and enduring eating disorders (SEED): certification, harm reduction, palliative care, and the question of futility. J Psychiatr Pract 2016;22(4):13–20.
19. Westmoreland P, Mehler PS. Ethical and medico-legal considerations in treating patients with eating disorders. In: Mehler PS, Andersen AE, editors. Eating disorders: a guide to medical care and complications. 3rd edition. Baltimore MD: John Hopkins University Press; 2017. p. 278–309.
20. Westmoreland P, Johnson C, Stafford M, Martinez R, Mehler PS. Involuntary treatment of patients with life-threatening anorexia nervosa. J Am Acad Psychiatry Law 2017;45(4):419–25.
21. Ward A, Ramsay R, Russell G, Treasure J. Follow-up mortality study of compulsorily treated patients with anorexia nervosa. Int J Eat Disord 2015;48(7):860–5.
22. Ramsey R, Treasure J. Treating anorexia nervosa: psychiatrists have mixed views on the use of terminal care for anorexia nervosa. BMJ 1996;312(7024):182.
23. Lopez A, Yager J, Feinstein RE. Medical futility and psychiatry: palliative care and hospice care as a last resort in the treatment of refractory anorexia nervosa. Int J Eat Disord 2010;43(4):372–7.
24. Campbell AT, Aulisio MP. The stigma of "mental" illness: end stage anorexia and treatment refusal. Int J Eat Disord 2012;45(5):627–34.
25. O'Neill J, Crowther T, Sampson G. Anorexia nervosa. Palliative care of terminal psychiatric disease. Am J Hosp Palliat Care 1994;11(6):36–8.
26. Local Authority v E. EWHC 1639, 2012.
27. Ryan CJ, Callaghan S. Treatment refusal in anorexia nervosa: the hardest cases. J Bioeth Inq 2014;11(1):43–5.
28. NHS Foundation Trust v. Ms X EWCOP 35, 2014.
29. Re Miss W EWCOP 13, 2016.
30. In the Matter of A.G., Incapacitated person, Superior court of New Jersey, MRS-P-1448-2016, 2016.
31. Jackson JZ. A case note regarding force-feeding of anorexic patients and the right to die. MD Advis 2017;10(4):21–4.
32. In the Matter of S.A. FH#2017-0039, 2017.
33. Kendall S. Anorexia nervosa: the diagnosis. J Bioethical Inq 2014;11:31–40.
34. Yager J. The futility of arguing about medical futility in anorexia nervosa: the question is how you would handle highly specific circumstances? Am J Bioeth 2015;15(7):47–50.
35. McKinney C. Is resistance (n)ever futile? A response to "Futility in chronic anorexia nervosa: a concept whose time has not yet come" by Cynthia Geppert. Am J Bioeth 2015;15(7):53–4.

Respect for Persons in the Psychiatric Treatment of Children and Adolescents

Rachel Conrad, MD[a],*, Bethany Brumbaugh, BA[b]

KEYWORDS

• Ethics • Child psychiatry • Adolescents • Medical decision making • Autonomy

KEY POINTS

- The clinical practice of child and adolescent psychiatry involves simultaneously balancing duties to various vulnerable parties.
- Respect for persons in the process of decision-making, particularly with adolescents, requires granting developmentally appropriate self-determination and privacy to the patient whenever possible
- The complexity of balancing these duties is often compounded when caring for intersectional populations facing inadequate access to mental health and psychosocial resources.
- The lack of evidence-based treatment recommendations, pervasive off-label use of medication, and increasing prescribing and polypharmacy in the most vulnerable patient populations are cause for concern about issues of equity in psychiatric care.

INTRODUCTION

The historical studies of hepatitis conducted among the children suffering from neuropsychiatric disorders at Willowbrook State School in the 1960s first brought to light many special considerations concerning vulnerability and care in child psychiatry.[1,2] The public debate following this controversial research, designed to study the course of hepatitis by deliberately infecting institutionalized minors, led to much of the current conceptualization of ethical duties in both pediatric clinical practice and pediatric research.[3,4]

Although aspects of child psychiatry have shifted during the intervening 6 decades, the contextual factors of inadequate services and resources in child psychiatry remain. For example, today, severe shortages of child psychiatrists affect most parts of the United States and lead to significant delays in care.[5–7] In addition, increasing rates of psychiatric disorders among children and inadequate access to outpatient

---

[a] Department of Psychiatry, Harvard Medical School, Harvard Medical School Center for Bioethics, Brigham and Women's Hospital, 221 Longwood Avenue, Boston, MA, USA; [b] Harvard Medical School, 25 Shattuck St, Boston, MA 02115, USA
* Corresponding author.
E-mail address: RConrad@BWH.Harvard.edu
Twitter: @DrRachelConrad (R.C.)

Psychiatr Clin N Am 44 (2021) 613–625
https://doi.org/10.1016/j.psc.2021.08.007
0193-953X/21/© 2021 Elsevier Inc. All rights reserved.

services often result in overuse of emergency departments for psychiatric services.[8,9] Many children in psychiatric crises are left boarding in emergency departments or pediatric hospital beds while waiting for mental health treatment.[10] Although it is undoubtedly ineffective, unsafe, and potentially traumatic, the boarding of children for psychiatric treatment appears to be increasing.[11] The families seeking services at Willowbrook State School were desperate to find care for their children, and many families continue to struggle with this challenge today. Distributive justice concerns regarding the quality of and access to psychiatric treatment for children are increasing as well. Many children do not receive evidence-based psychotherapy when needed, and inappropriate psychopharmacologic practices are pervasive.[12–15] Child psychiatrists struggle to maintain the safety of the child and family against this backdrop of inadequate services and systems.

The clinical practice of child and adolescent psychiatry involves simultaneously balancing duties toward various vulnerable parties: children with psychiatric illness and their often distressed families. The care of children involves the complex dynamics of the physician-patient-parent relationship as the rights and obligations of each are weighed throughout the treatment of the child.[16] Balancing autonomy and protection within the psychiatric treatment of adolescents is particularly complex, and state laws governing these issues often add further confusion. Child and adolescent psychiatry will continue to encounter various concerns that challenge the rights, preferences, and duties to persons and families.

DECISION MAKING

Respect for persons requires that individuals should be treated as autonomous agents when possible, and those with diminished capacity are entitled to protection.[17] As a result, regardless of whether children have legal rights to medical decision making, as an ethical imperative they should be granted developmentally appropriate self-determination and privacy whenever possible.[18] A child or adolescent's decision-making capacity depends on multiple, complex interactions between their age, psychosocial development, maturity, intellectual ability, neuropsychiatric presentation, and the specific decision at hand.[19–21] In general, by ages 12 to 14 years, most children demonstrate mastery of the core skills involved in medical decision making: understanding of their situation, appreciation of the consequences, reasoning about their options, and expression of a choice.[22] After studies showed that adolescents demonstrate capacity for informed decision making, many states expanded legal rights of adolescents, and professional codes advocated for the involvement of adolescents in medical decision making.[23,24]

To help clinicians navigate questions of decision-making capacity in children, the American Academy of Pediatrics Committee on Bioethics introduced the paired concepts of parental permission and patient assent in 1995 following a decade of deliberation.[25] Their statement championed "the experience, perspective and power of children" and required that children participate in decision making commensurate with their development and provide assent to care whenever possible. The ethical standards published by the American Academy of Pediatrics include transparency with children about diagnostic and treatment interventions and allowing children to have choices about aspects of their care.[26] Furthermore, a pediatric patient's dissent should carry considerable weight, including that the unwanted intervention be deferred when not urgent or essential. Appropriately engaging children in medical decision making may have added positive effects of fostering their moral growth, maturity, and development.[25] Psychiatric treatment outcomes are optimal when the patient, family, and physician all actively engage in both the decision-making process and the treatment in a developmentally appropriate manner, starting in childhood and extending through young adulthood.[27] The engagement of all parties increases treatment adherence and supports children to gradually build skills to navigate their own medical care.

Child and adolescent psychiatrists also benefit from attunement to their own values and views about treatment decisions for their patients as research shows that physicians caring for pediatric patients tend to selectively grant a pediatric patient decision-making capacity and input when the patient's decision aligns with the physician's opinion of the patient's best interest.[28] This feature of the doctor-patient interaction raises awareness of the need for clarity and transparency in medical decision making for minors. For example, the American Academy of Pediatrics considers any deception during the process of assessing decision-making capacity and assent unethical and cautions that patients should not be deceived by either physicians or parents during their medical care.[26] In practice, in situations when an intervention is judged to be imperative by both the physician and the parents, and the patient will not be allowed any choice in treatment limitation or refusal, the child should be informed about the decision and their preference not elicited if it will not be seriously considered. Respect for the child requires transparency and honesty in the reasons for soliciting preferences and avoiding situations in which preferences are solicited even though the treatment team has no intent to consider those preferences. Similarly, only granting a child or adolescent input in medical decisions when the patient's choices align with the preferences of others falls short of respecting patient autonomy.

INVOLUNTARY TREATMENT

As in the treatment of adults, certain clinical circumstances in which an individual poses a risk of harm to self or others owing to mental illness may result in limiting the autonomy of a child or adolescent. One extreme of loss of patient autonomy in children, adolescents, and adults is the use of involuntary treatment and/or restraints.[29] However, the justifications and reasoning that guide involuntary treatment of children and adolescents extend beyond the adult corollary. Because of the critical developmental and growth period that occurs early in life, the effects of neuropsychiatric illness have the potential to set the physical and mental health trajectory for the entirety of a child's life. For example, substance use during adolescence is associated with an array of short- and long-term consequences, including depressive disorders, psychotic disorders, impaired executive functioning, lower academic achievement, physically and sexually risky behavior, violence, and suicide.[30] Eating disorders during adolescence are associated with stunted growth, osteoporosis, psychiatric disorders, substance use, starvation, suicide, and alarming increase in all-cause mortality.[31] The patient's best-interest standard and questionable competency in refusing beneficial treatments for conditions associated with elevated mortality rate may justify the infringement of autonomy to force or coerce children in certain circumstances owing to the long-term potential for harm. These rationales, in essence, on balance favor the weight of beneficence and nonmaleficence over autonomy.

However, involuntary treatment is not without harm: it is distressing and potentially traumatic for patients, their family, and, often, the clinicians and staff involved. Even when involuntary measures, force, or coercion is beneficial in improving short-term physical health outcomes, the long-term psychological and developmental impact on the patient must be considered.[32] Two hypotheses have guided researchers who study involuntary treatment: the first is that force angers patients, engrains a negative attitude about their care during the treatment, and thereby causes further psychological problems and reduced willingness to engage in treatment in the long term; the second, opposing, view is that the initial negativity will give way to acceptance, positivity, willing engagement, and consequently lead to the reduction of symptoms.[32] The longitudinal data to support either of these perspectives are mixed and remain controversial, especially in the context of adolescents, who, as they grapple with many rapid changes and approach the transition to adulthood are vulnerable to feelings of disempowerment.[33] Therefore, removing their ability to meaningfully participate in decisions about their own medical care may damage self-esteem, self-efficacy, and future ability to navigate medical decisions.

Finally, although state laws, professional societies, and institutions often generate recommendations about the patient's rights and duties in a medical decision-making process, a decision within a family is not made in a vacuum. True voluntariness in a decision by either parents or children is unrealistic as fundamental interdependence influences the medical decision-making process.[34] The nature of shared resources and circumstances within family life often extends into young adulthood, beyond the age when a patient is legally granted the right to independent medical decision making.[35]

BEST-INTEREST STANDARD

Legal standards for a parent to act as the default medical decision maker for their own child are driven by assumptions about parents' intrinsic motivation to act in the best interest of their child. Notable cases, such as the studies at the Willowbrook State School and the US Supreme Court case *Parham v JR*, identified and brought to light circumstances in which parents sought treatment driven by external circumstances that may not have been in the best interest of their own child, often pertaining to involuntary psychiatric hospitalization or institutionalization of a child.[36] As a result, the American Academy of Pediatrics has reframed the discussion about pediatric decision making from the parents' rights to autonomous decisions to the parents' duty to support the best interest of their child.[26] The best-interest standard aims to maximize benefits and minimize harm to the minor; however, it has been criticized as vague.[37–39] Another approach from the perspective of the harm principle is used to identify parental decisions that will not be tolerated because of the physicians' duty to protect the child.[40] More recent frameworks have shifted to balance the patient's emotional, social, and medical concerns with the interests of the family.[26] In the end, even with clarity that the child's or adolescent's welfare is paramount, significant challenges persist in determining what, exactly, constitutes fulfilment of this ethical and legal responsibility.

ADOLESCENT DECISION MAKING

As adolescents have increasing capacity to appropriately reason through medical decisions, encouraging them to engage in these processes promotes respect for their autonomy and self-determination, and efforts to do so therefore are autonomy promoting.[41,42] During late adolescence, when an adolescent's wishes are known to a physician and family, substituted judgment, that is, making decisions in accordance what the adolescent would want if competent to consent, should replace the best-interest standard to guide decision making on behalf of an adolescent.[26] In other words, as the child matures into adolescence, the relative priority of their voice increases over what others judge to be best for them.

In a limited but generally well-delineated set of circumstances, the ability of minors to make decisions on their own behalf in combination with features of their lives and/or public policy considerations has led to the emergence of laws recognizing their right to do so. Specifically, minors are granted legal rights to medical decision making in a range of circumstances that vary widely by state.[24,43] In general, "emancipated minors" are granted decisional rights based on their social circumstances, regardless of age, such as living independently, being self-supporting, being married, parenting their own children, or serving in the military.[44] A second category of adolescents, "mature minors," are permitted to make decisions in certain clinical situations owing to one of several factors, including age, maturity, cognitive abilities, and circumstances, including treatment of certain stigmatized conditions.[26] These conditions include pregnancy, sexually transmitted disease, substance use, and psychiatric disorders, and minors may be able to consent to treatment for these conditions without parental consent as young as age 12.[45]

State laws governing the age of consent for psychiatric and substance use treatment often seem arbitrary and confusing to physicians.[24,46] In addition to inconsistencies between states, many states have conflicting laws governing psychotherapy and psychopharmacologic treatment, inpatient and outpatient settings, psychiatric and substance use disorders, and issues of consent and privacy.[24,43,44] Many states allow minors to consent to substance use treatment but not to other forms of mental health treatment, and the reason for this disparity is unclear, although it may be related to the stigma of substance use, the importance of seeking treatment, and fear of a punitive rather than a rehabilitative parental response.[24] Twenty-four states have laws allowing adolescent access to treatment but do not specify an age of consent.[46] Most states' laws do not address the course of action when a parent and child disagree about the need for treatment.[43] In sum, the presence of mature minor laws are an important example of the indeterminate nature of the ability to consent based on age, especially in late adolescence. The ethical importance of respecting the adolescent's preferences in treatment decisions as an autonomy-promoting matter and in consideration of what course of action should be taken in the patient's interest, on balance, can serve as a steady guide.

SUBSTANCE USE DISORDERS

Adolescent substance use has a range of long-term consequences, and alarmingly few adolescents receive adequate treatment for substance use disorders. In efforts to increase access to substance use treatment among adolescents, 44 states now allow minors to consent to substance use treatment without their parents' consent.[47] However, in consideration of care and nonmaleficence responsibilities, it is also important to recognize that parental collaboration is critical to effective substance use treatment, and it is unclear if allowing minors to consent for substance use treatment without their parental involvement meaningfully improves either access or outcomes.[24] Furthermore, some argue that rather than expanding an adolescent's right to decision making in the context of a substance use disorder, the adolescent's right to decision making should actually be restricted because of the impaired judgment caused by substance use. Although the adolescent's substance use impacts their own long-term neuropsychiatric functioning, active substance use impacts family members, and the duties to the family may be considered.

There is widespread confusion about the clinical implications of these laws, and many physicians feel unprepared to address these issues clinically.[24,48] As psychiatric and substance use disorders typically cooccur and their treatments are intrinsically intertwined, clinicians are perplexed when the age of consent differs between psychiatric and substance use treatments. Furthermore, some state laws specify that an adolescent is entitled to autonomous medical decision making without parental consent but do not address whether the adolescent is entitled to privacy. Experts express concerns that the laws governing adolescent consent for substance use are not guided by scientific research or clinical rationale.[24,46,49] Further empirical study could help advance evidence-based decisional paradigms and inform ethical approaches to these dilemmas.

EATING DISORDERS

Ethical dilemmas regarding involuntary treatment and coercion arise commonly in eating disorder treatment.[50,51] Although similar dilemmas occur within eating disorder treatment across the lifespan, additional considerations and duties must be considered when encountering children and adolescents with eating disorders as compared with adults. One set of responsibilities stems from protective responsibilities related to children's and adolescents' membership in a vulnerable group of persons. In addition, broad developmental considerations encompassing present and future well-being play prominently. For example, compromised nutritional status within a critical developmental period can lead to both swift health deterioration and long-term medical consequences, such as stunted growth, osteopenia, and infertility.[52] Efforts to reduce the risk of developing a chronic eating disorder may also justify involuntary treatment earlier in the presentation of disordered eating.[53] In addition to the inherently reduced autonomy and lack of true voluntariness, the duty to protect often overrides the patient's autonomy in treatment of children and adolescents with eating disorders.

Determination of competency in patients with eating disorders is complex across the lifespan. Current concepts of capacity and standard tests of competence may be inadequate to identify and/or assess the decision-making abilities of patients with eating disorders.[54] Even if judged to be competent through standard metrics, treatment refusal may be considered a symptom of the disease, and deteriorating health has been considered an indication that the patient does not understand the implications of treatment refusal.[55] In contrast to adults, children may not be able to adequately comprehend the long-term consequences of an eating disorder because of limited life experience and their development stage.

Involuntary hospitalization and nasogastric tube feeding of patients experiencing acute medical decompensation represent extreme loss of autonomy for patients with eating disorders. However, more subtle intrusion and coercion are pervasive within eating disorder treatments and should be both recognized and ethically justified. Common interventions in eating disorder treatment include exercise restriction, surveillance of meals, surveillance of bathrooms, forced pharmacotherapy, and restrictions of activity and visitors based on compliance to treatment.[51] Methods involving coercion and inducement in eating disorder treatment are criticized by some as inherently unethical while often necessary to promote the safety of patients. Although involuntary treatment may be beneficial for acute medical stabilization, little evidence supports the long-term efficacy of involuntary and coercive treatment for adolescents with eating disorders.[33]

Especially given the unclear long-term impact and the danger of framing coercive and intrusive practices in treatment within the duty to care, patient autonomy remains an important consideration. In other words, the duty to protect, forced treatment, and coercion are all important considerations in the context of individual patients, with every effort being made to engage the adolescent as an active participant.

CONFIDENTIALITY

Conflicts around privacy and confidentiality, particularly involving stigmatized and high-risk behaviors among adolescents, are complex.[56–58] Most physicians across specialties report feeling unprepared to navigate confidentiality laws pertaining to adolescents.[48] Federal and state laws addressing minors' right to privacy are often confusing; for example, many states that allow minors to consent for treatment do not explicitly provide the right to privacy.[26]

Physicians confronted with a decision about breaking a child or adolescent's confidentiality by disclosing information to a parent must weigh the potential benefits versus the harms and consider what is in the child's best interest.[59] A significant potential harm associated with disclosing information to a patients' parents is the damage to the psychotherapeutic relationship. It is critical to first explore with the child or adolescent patient what negative consequences are anticipated from the parental disclosure. The safety of the parent-child relationship, the likelihood of a problematic, punitive, or even abusive reaction to the information, and other potential harms resulting from the disclosure must be seriously considered. If a disclosure remains justified despite thorough consideration of potential harms, the physician then must help the patient understand their justification for the disclosure and make efforts to preserve rapport and the therapeutic relationship to avoid collateral harms. Ideally, the physician and patient will collaborate with the goal that the patient will provide permission for the disclosure, and both the patient and the physician will engage in the conversation with the parent or parents together.

As the prevalence of both cannabis and nicotine use has recently increased among adolescents, decisions about whether to inform parents about a child or adolescent patient's substance use are increasingly common.[60] The National Advisory Council on Drug Abuse has advised that sensitive information, including the use of illegal drugs by persons under the age of 18, should not be disclosed to parents unless there is a risk of imminent danger to the patient or someone else.[61] However, risk of imminent danger is vague and subjective. Pragmatically, if substance use is frequent and severe enough to place a patient at imminent risk of danger, the parents are typically already aware.[62] The increasing patient and family access to the electronic medical records now highlights the reality of the risk of inadvertent disclosure about confidential information obtained during treatment.[41]

SOCIAL CONTEXT OF FUNCTIONAL IMPAIRMENT

Criteria for psychiatric diagnoses often rest on the functional impairment caused by the symptoms. In child psychiatry, functional impairment is typically based on subjective reports by parents, teachers, and other adults. Degree of impairment from the symptoms is often further affected by external factors, including stressors, resources, and the ability of the adult to understand and manage the child's feelings and behavior.

Relying on subjective reports of others sometimes interferes with psychiatric care. For example, children who are the youngest in their class are more than twice as likely as their peers to be diagnosed with attention-deficit/hyperactivity disorder (ADHD) and treated with a stimulant, likely because gaps in performance and behavior owing to relative biological immaturity are misinterpreted as psychiatric symptoms.[63–65] Peculiarities of context and misunderstandings among the adults who are reporting the symptoms can lead to misdiagnosis and inappropriate treatment in certain circumstances.

Some families struggle to manage developmentally appropriate behaviors because of social circumstances and resource limitations. Certain parent-child interaction styles exacerbate attentional, emotional, and behavioral symptoms among children.[66,67] Families living in poverty experience chronic stress, and the myriad challenges of life in poverty frequently interfere with effective parenting and fostering a developmentally appropriate home environment. In addition, families living in poverty often lack access to adequate childcare, education, nutrition, physical activity, and other resources critical to the healthy development of a child, which leads to a range of chronic medical conditions.[68] These factors may exacerbate a child's psychiatric symptoms or interfere with appropriate diagnosis and treatment as well. For example, complaints about impulsive behavior or inattention may stem from inadequate child-care when a child simply needs structure and adult supervision. Exercise is well known to help manage symptoms of ADHD, and ADHD may be exacerbated when children lack access to sports, physical education, and outdoor activities.[69] These external limitations within the child's environment may lead to the use of stimulants and other psychotropic medications to treat relatively mild symptoms that could be managed with appropriate psychosocial resources and would not cause impairment in another context.

Childhood poverty may also contribute to adverse childhood experiences, which are linked to a range of long-term medical and psychiatric outcomes.[70] However, targeted interventions can reduce the risk of psychiatric disorders among children who grow up in poverty. For example, evidence-based social-emotional learning programs during preschool can lead to significant long-term benefits, including decreased conduct problems, emotional symptoms, and peer problems during adolescence.[71] Unfortunately, these programs are often unavailable because of inadequate funding.

Antipsychotic use among children living in foster care provides an example of how the interaction between the child, their stressors, and their environment may lead to inappropriate prescribing of psychotropic medication. Children in foster care are prescribed psychotropics at alarmingly high rates, often in the absence of a psychiatric diagnosis that justifies their treatment.[72] Although interventions in child psychiatry must often balance the needs of the patients with others in their environment to maintain everyone's safety, inappropriate prescribing without the implementation of appropriate psychosocial interventions violates ethical duties to the child.

DIAGNOSIS AND TREATMENT WITH PSYCHOTROPIC MEDICATION

Off-label prescribing is pervasive within the clinical practice of child psychiatry, and many psychotropic medications lack adequate data about long-term safety and efficacy in children and adolescents. The ethics of psychiatric research in children is complex, and the barriers to research of psychotropic medication in children are manifold.[4,73] As the incidence of psychiatric illness among children increases, research that establishes psychotropic medications' long-term safety and efficacy in children is critical. Inadequate psychotropic research in children forces physicians to weigh the effects of chronic psychopathology against unknown long-term adverse effects of psychopharmacologic treatment.[74] Psychiatric research on children and adolescents is ethically justified by the need to reduce the burden that mental illnesses place on young people, their families, and society.[75]

Many common prescribing patterns in child psychiatry lack robust evidence, and utilization of stimulants, atypical antipsychotics, and polypharmacy has skyrocketed in recent decades. Although atypical antipsychotics have concerning adverse effect profiles, the use of atypical antipsychotics to treat ADHD, disruptive behaviors in children without autism, and mood problems in children without bipolar disorder has increased, despite limited efficacy for these conditions.[72,76] One study found that one-third of children in foster care were simultaneously prescribed 2 atypical antipsychotics for more than 3 months, a prescribing practice that lacks empirical research for efficacy in children and is associated with significant increased risk of metabolic adverse effects.[72]

Finally, significant justice concerns arise from alarming patterns in both psychiatric diagnoses and treatment of children of color and children in legal or state custody.[77,78] Boys are much more likely to be diagnosed with ADHD than girls, leading to concerns of overdiagnosis in boys and underrecognition in girls.[63] Black children are much more likely to be prescribed an antipsychotic than white children. Children in foster care are much more likely to be diagnosed with bipolar disorder and are prescribed atypical antipsychotics at unusually high rates. Inappropriate overprescribing of antipsychotics may function as a chemical restraint to sedate children rather than devoting adequate psychosocial resources and evidence-based psychotherapeutic interventions.

FUTURE DIRECTIONS

Ethical dilemmas commonly arise while navigating competing duties to the child, parents, family, and community in the clinical practice of child and adolescent psychiatry. Addressing these dilemmas with developmentally appropriate communication and collaborative decision making with the child and family is critical. Principles of both justice and respect for persons require the availability of safe, adequate, and appropriate psychiatric treatment for all children. Psychotropic medication should be guided by empirical research and not misused to manage behavioral issues that would be more appropriately addressed by psychosocial interventions.

Social determinants of health, health care disparities, lack of access, and inappropriate prescribing to members of vulnerable and intersectional populations are increasingly receiving well-justified attention in both the academic literature and the popular press. Ethical duties in child psychiatry demand access to evidence-based psychotherapy, social services, community resources, and educational systems, all of which are critical to promoting the mental health of children.

CLINICS CARE POINTS

- Children and adolescents should be granted developmentally appropriate self-determination and privacy whenever possible regardless of their legal rights to medical decision making.

- For children who are not able to engage in medical decision making because of their developmental stage, the best-interest standard and harm principle should guide treatment decisions.

- Minors are granted legal rights to consent to mental health and substance use treatment in a range of clinical and psychosocial situations, which vary widely by state.

- Social determinants of health may exacerbate a child's psychiatric symptoms and interfere with appropriate treatment.

- Significant concerns about distributive justice arise from alarming patterns in psychiatric care of children of color and children in legal or state custody.

- Safe and appropriate use of psychotropic medications as well as psychosocial interventions is critical for ethical psychiatric care of children.

DISCLOSURE

The authors have nothing to disclose.

REFERENCES

1. Beecher HK. Ethics and clinical research. N Engl J Med 1966;274(24):1354–60.
2. Robinson W. The hepatitis experiments at the Willowbrook State School. The oxford textbook of clinical research ethics. Oxford; New York: Oxford University Press; 2008.
3. Litton P. Non-beneficial pediatric research and the best interests standard: a legal and ethical reconciliation. Yale J Health Policy Law Ethics 2008;8(2):359–420.
4. Gandhi R. Research involving children: regulations, review boards and reform. J Health Care Law Policy 2005;8(2):264–330.
5. Cama S, Malowney M, Smith AJB, et al. Availability of outpatient mental health care by pediatricians and child psychiatrists in five U.S. cities. Int J Health Serv 2017;47(4):621–35.
6. Malowney M, Keltz S, Fischer D, et al. Availability of outpatient care from psychiatrists: a simulated-patient study in three U.S. cities. Psychiatr Serv 2015; 66(1):94–6.
7. Beck A, Page C, Buche J, et al. Estimating the Distribution of the U.S. Psychiatric Subspecialist Workforce. Ann Arbor, MI: University of Michigan School of Public Health; 2018.
8. Nicks BA, Manthey DM. The impact of psychiatric patient boarding in emergency departments. Emerg Med Int 2012;2012:360308.
9. Nordstrom K, Berlin JS, Nash SS, et al. Boarding of mentally ill patients in emergency departments: American Psychiatric Association resource document. West J Emerg Med 2019;20(5):690–5.
10. Rabin E, Kocher K, McClelland M, et al. Solutions to emergency department 'boarding' and crowding are underused and may need to be legislated. Health Aff (Millwood) 2012;31(8):1757–66.
11. McEnany FB, Ojugbele O, Doherty JR, et al. Pediatric mental health boarding. Pediatrics 2020;146(4):e20201174.
12. Rettew DC, Greenblatt J, Kamon J, et al. Antipsychotic medication prescribing in children enrolled in Medicaid. Pediatrics 2015;135(4):658–65.
13. Pathak P, West D, Martin BC, et al. Evidence-based use of second-generation antipsychotics in a state Medicaid pediatric population, 2001-2005. Psychiatr Serv 2010;61(2):123–9.
14. Burcu M, Zito JM, Ibe A, et al. Atypical antipsychotic use among Medicaid-insured children and adolescents: duration, safety, and monitoring implications. J Child Adolesc Psychopharmacol 2014;24(3):112–9.
15. Girand HL, Litkowiec S, Sohn M. Attention-deficit/hyperactivity disorder and psychotropic polypharmacy prescribing trends. Pediatrics 2020;146(1):e20192832.
16. Cummings CL, Mercurio MR. Ethics for the pediatrician: autonomy, beneficence, and rights. Pediatr Rev 2010;31(6):252–5.
17. National Commission for the Protection of Human Subjects of Biomedical and Behavioral Research. The Belmont report: ethical principles and guidelines for the protection of human subjects of research. Bethesda, MD. 1976.
18. Mercurio MR, Maxwell MA, Mears BJ, et al. American Academy of Pediatrics Policy Statements on bioethics: summaries and commentaries: part 2. Pediatr Rev 2008;29(3):e15–22.
19. Weithorn LA, Campbell SB. The competency of children and adolescents to make informed treatment decisions. Child Dev 1982;53(6):1589–98.
20. Appelbaum PS, Grisso T. Assessing patients' capacities to consent to treatment. N Engl J Med 1988;319(25):1635–8.

21. Grisso T, Vierling L. Minors' consent to treatment: a developmental perspective. Prof Psychol 1978;9(3):412–27.
22. Hein IM, Troost PW, Lindeboom R, et al. Accuracy of the MacArthur Competence Assessment Tool for Clinical Research (MacCAT-CR) for measuring children's competence to consent to clinical research. JAMA Pediatr 2014;168(12):1147.
23. Poncz E. Rethinking child advocacy after Ropver v. Simmons: "kids are just different" and "kids are like adults" advocacy strategies. Cardoza Public Law Pol Ethics J 2008;6(2):273–343.
24. Kerwin ME, Kirby KC, Speziali D, et al. What can parents do? A review of state laws regarding decision making for adolescent drug abuse and mental health treatment. J Child Adolesc Subst Abuse 2015;24(3):166–76.
25. Informed consent, parental permission, and assent in pediatric practice. Committee on Bioethics, American Academy of Pediatrics. Pediatrics 1995;95(2):314–7.
26. Informed consent in decision-making in pediatric practice. Pediatrics 2016; 138(2):e20161484.
27. Family-centered care and the pediatrician's role. Pediatrics 2003;112(3 Pt 1): 691–7.
28. de Vries MC, Bresters D, Engberts DP, et al. Attitudes of physicians and parents towards discussing infertility risks and semen cryopreservation with male adolescents diagnosed with cancer. Pediatr Blood Cancer 2009;53(3):386–91.
29. Geng F, Jiang F, Conrad R, et al. Factors associated with involuntary psychiatric hospitalization of youths in China based on a nationally representative sample. Front Psychiatry 2020;11:607464.
30. Cho H, Hallfors DD, Iritani BJ. Early initiation of substance use and subsequent risk factors related to suicide among urban high school students. Addict Behav 2007;32(8):1628–39.
31. Errichiello L, Iodice D, Bruzzese D, et al. Prognostic factors and outcome in anorexia nervosa: a follow-up study. Eat Weight Disord 2016;21(1):73–82.
32. Hiday VA. Involuntary commitment as a psychiatric technology. Int J Technol Assess Health Care 1996;12(4):585–603.
33. Elzakkers IF, Danner UN, Hoek HW, et al. Compulsory treatment in anorexia nervosa: a review. Int J Eat Disord 2014;47(8):845–52.
34. Lipstein EA, Brinkman WB, Britto MT. What is known about parents' treatment decisions? A narrative review of pediatric decision making. Med Decis Making 2012;32(2):246–58.
35. Conrad R. Legal and ethical challenges in the psychiatric treatment of college students. Curr Psychiatry Rep 2020;22(9):50.
36. Redding RE. Children's competence to provide informed consent for mental health treatment. Wash Lee Law Rev 1993;50(2):695–753.
37. Kopelman LM. The best-interests standard as threshold, ideal, and standard of reasonableness. J Med Philos 1997;22(3):271–89.
38. Veatch RM. Abandoning informed consent. Hastings Cent Rep 1995;25(2):5–12.
39. Bester JC. The best interest standard is the best we have: why the harm principle and constrained parental autonomy cannot replace the best interest standard in pediatric ethics. J Clin Ethics 2019;30(3):223–31.
40. Diekema D. Parental refusals of medical treatment: the harm principle as threshold for state intervention. Theor Med Bioeth 2004;25(4):243–64.
41. Berlan ED, Bravender T. Confidentiality, consent, and caring for the adolescent patient. Curr Opin Pediatr 2009;21(4):450–6.
42. Hickey K. Minors' rights in medical decision making. JONAS Healthc Law Ethics Regul 2007;9(3):100–4 [quiz 105–6].

43. Lallemont T, Mastroianni A, Wickizer TM. Decision-making authority and substance abuse treatment for adolescents: a survey of state laws. J Adolesc Health 2009;44(4):323–34.
44. Fortunati FG Jr, Zonana HV. Legal considerations in the child psychiatric emergency department. Child Adolesc Psychiatr Clin N Am 2003;12(4):745–61.
45. English A. Understanding legal aspects of care. Adolescent health care: a practical guide. 5th edition. New York: Walters Kluwer/Lippincott Williams & Wilkins; 2008.
46. Weisleder P. Inconsistency among American states on the age at which minors can consent to substance abuse treatment. J Am Acad Psychiatry Law 2007; 35(3):317–22.
47. Ford C, English A, Sigman G. Confidential health care for adolescents: position paper for the Society for Adolescent Medicine. J Adolesc Health 2004;35(2): 160–7.
48. Riley M, Ahmed S, Reed BD, et al. Physician knowledge and attitudes around confidential care for minor patients. J Pediatr Adolesc Gynecol 2015;28(4):234–9.
49. Meyer DJ. Commentary: legislators how did the deciders decide? Who shall serve as their experts? J Am Acad Psychiatry Law 2007;35(3):323–4.
50. Macdonald C. Treatment resistance in anorexia nervosa and the pervasiveness of ethics in clinical decision making. Can J Psychiatry 2002;47(3):267–70.
51. Matusek JA, Wright MO. Ethical dilemmas in treating clients with eating disorders: a review and application of an integrative ethical decision-making model. Eur Eat Disord Rev 2010;18(6):434–52.
52. Manley RS, Smye V, Srikameswaran S. Addressing complex ethical issues in the treatment of children and adolescents with eating disorders: application of a framework for ethical decision-making. Eur Eat Disord Rev 2001;9(3):144–66.
53. Carney T, Tait D, Touyz S, et al. Managing anorexia nervosa: clinical, legal and social perspectives on involuntary treatment. In: Managing anorexia nervosa: clinical, legal and social perspectives on involuntary treatment. Nova Science Publishers; 2006. p. vii, 195–vii, 195.
54. Tan J, Hope T, Stewart A. Competence to refuse treatment in anorexia nervosa. Int J L Psychiatry 2003;26(6):697–707.
55. Doig C, Burgess E. Withholding life-sustaining treatment: are adolescents competent to make these decisions? CMAJ 2000;162(11):1585–8.
56. Sullivan JR, Ramirez E, Rae WA, et al. Factors contributing to breaking confidentiality with adolescent clients: a survey of pediatric psychologists. Prof Psychol Res Pract 2002;33(4):396–401.
57. Koocher GP. Ethical challenges in mental health services to children and families. J Clin Psychol 2008;64(5):601–12.
58. Maslyanskaya S, Alderman EM. Confidentiality and consent in the care of the adolescent patient. Pediatr Rev 2019;40(10):508–16.
59. Taylor L, Adelman HS. Reframing the confidentiality dilemma to work in children's best interests. Prof Psychol Res Pract 1989;20(2):79–83.
60. Rosales A. Conflicting ethics of confidentiality in adolescent drug research. Psychopharmacology (Berl) 2014;231(8):1433.
61. National Advisory Council on Drug Abuse. National Advisory Council on Drug Abuse guidelines for substance abuse research involving children and adolescents. Bethesda, MD; Department of Health and Human Services; 2005.
62. Dougherty DM, Hill-Kapturczak N, Ryan SR, et al. Ethical considerations in adolescent drug research. Psychopharmacology (Berl) 2014;231(8):1433–5.

63. Te Meerman S, Batstra L, Grietens H, et al. ADHD: a critical update for educational professionals. Int J Qual Stud Health Well-being 2017;12(sup1):1298267.
64. Evans WN, Morrill MS, Parente ST. Measuring inappropriate medical diagnosis and treatment in survey data: the case of ADHD among school-age children. J Health Econ 2010;29(5):657–73.
65. Zoëga H, Valdimarsdóttir UA, Hernández-Díaz S. Age, academic performance, and stimulant prescribing for ADHD: a nationwide cohort study. Pediatrics 2012;130(6):1012–8.
66. Kissgen R, Franke S. An attachment research perspective on ADHD. Neuropsychiatrie 2016;30(2):63–8.
67. Teixeira MC, Marino RL, Carreiro LR. Associations between inadequate parenting practices and behavioral problems in children and adolescents with attention deficit hyperactivity disorder. ScientificWorldJournal 2015;2015:683062.
68. Pulcini CD, Zima BT, Kelleher KJ, et al. Poverty and trends in three common chronic disorders. Pediatrics 2017;139(3):e20162539.
69. Song M, Lauseng D, Lee S, et al. Enhanced physical activity improves selected outcomes in children with ADHD: systematic review. West J Nurs Res 2016;38(9):1155–84.
70. Mersky JP, Topitzes J, Reynolds AJ. Impacts of adverse childhood experiences on health, mental health, and substance use in early adulthood: a cohort study of an urban, minority sample in the U.S. Child Abuse Negl 2013;37(11):917–25.
71. Bierman KL, Heinrichs BS, Welsh JA, et al. Reducing adolescent psychopathology in socioeconomically disadvantaged children with a preschool intervention: a randomized controlled trial. Am J Psychiatry 2020. https://doi.org/10.1176/appi.ajp.2020.20030343.
72. Dosreis S, Yoon Y, Rubin DM, et al. Antipsychotic treatment among youth in foster care. Pediatrics 2011;128(6):e1459–66.
73. Fleishman A, Collogan L. Chapter 42: research with children MsoNormal style: 150%. The Oxford textbook of clinical research ethics. Oxford; New York: Oxford University Press; 2008.
74. Vitiello B, Jensen PS. Medication development and testing in children and adolescents. Current problems, future directions. Arch Gen Psychiatry 1997;54(9):871–6.
75. Hoop JG, Smyth AC, Roberts LW. Ethical issues in psychiatric research on children and adolescents. Child Adolesc Psychiatr Clin N Am 2008;17(1):127–48, x.
76. Daviss WB, Barnett E, Neubacher K, et al. Use of antipsychotic medications for nonpsychotic children: risks and implications for mental health services. Psychiatr Serv 2016;67(3):339–41.
77. Simon KM. Them and me - the care and treatment of black boys in America. N Engl J Med 2020;383(20):1904–5.
78. Fadus MC, Ginsburg KR, Sobowale K, et al. Unconscious bias and the diagnosis of disruptive behavior disorders and ADHD in African American and Hispanic youth. Acad Psychiatry 2020;44(1):95–102.

Ethical Practice in Emergency Psychiatry
Common Dilemmas and Virtue-Informed Navigation

Brandon Hamm, MD, MS

KEYWORDS

- Emergency psychiatry • Bioethics • Virtue ethics • Involuntary commitment
- Agitation • Collateral information

KEY POINTS

- Ethical dilemmas in emergency psychiatry can arise due to conflicts between duties of care and protection of patients (parens patriae) or the safety of others (state police power).
- Obtaining nonconsensual collateral information is permissible and expected when necessary for psychiatric emergency care, and minimal disclosure is permissible to facilitate these conversations.
- Humane agitation management with respect for patient experience features graded implementation of least-invasive interventions, clear message of prevention and protection rather than punishment, and sincere communication including a debriefing.
- Virtues can provide holistic guidance for moral action in psychiatric emergencies where ethical principles conflict

INTRODUCTION

Emergency psychiatrists regularly encounter ethical dilemmas, and this article considers approaches that may promote and enhance ethics-informed practice in emergency situations. Although a checklist of rules to follow is likely be insufficient when navigating each unique situation that an emergency psychiatrist might face in day-to-day practice, an understanding of ethical moorings and the legal context of practice can inform sound practice balancing the often-complex needs of patients, as well as societal interests. Supplementing legal rules and ethical principles with guidance from ethical virtues may further promote more humane and holistic care in acute psychiatric settings. Specific examples described in this article include collecting collateral information, acute agitation management, medical clearance evaluation, involuntary holds, reporting of abuse and neglect, and warning and protecting third parties. Although

Northwestern University, 676 N St Clair St, 11th Floor, Chicago, IL 60611, USA
E-mail address: brandon.hamm@northwestern.edu

Psychiatr Clin N Am 44 (2021) 627–640
https://doi.org/10.1016/j.psc.2021.08.011
psych.theclinics.com

decision-making capacity and informed consent are essential for ethical practice in any clinical context, a detailed review of these topics is deferred in this review, but is delineated elsewhere regarding the emergency psychiatry context[1] as well as addressed in this issue in the Article , "Ethical Issues in Consultation-Liaison Psychiatry".

ADVANCING PRACTICE THROUGH INTEGRATION OF VIRTUE ETHICS INTO EMERGENCY PSYCHIATRIC PRACTICE

In the practice of psychiatry and medicine, clinical-ethical challenges arise when important values come into tension. In a multicultural, increasingly diverse profession, physicians are faced with balancing between competing clinical, ethical, and legal demands; concerns and ethical dilemmas often distill to choosing the least-worst option or following institutional and/or legal policy and/or precedent.[2] Ethical treatment in high-stakes emergency settings can advance beyond the sole balancing of competing ethical and legal interests in these settings, with additional attention toward qualities and character of psychiatrists as they strive to achieve the highest possible levels of professionalism, care, and wisdom. This approach to the character and quality of the moral agent is at the core of virtue ethics.

In The Nicomachean Ethics, Aristotle describes the process of phronesis (practical wisdom), whereby a person evaluates a context and makes judgments to determine moral action and virtues for application in the circumstance.[3,4] Right action is defined as what a virtuous person acting in accordance with virtue would do, or what a "good" doctor or psychiatrist would do is what a moral exemplar (or virtuous) physician would do in the same circumstances.[5] Virtue ethics directs focus on how to be rather than what to do; what to do is determined by what a virtuous person would do. As such, the focus of virtue ethics, like core aspects of professional development, is on developing the attitudes, skills, values, and temperament that lead one to act ethically. Radden and Sadler[6] propose that the unique duties of a psychiatrist, including the concomitant duties for patient care and public protection, may require a standard for virtuous practice beyond that of many other professions. Habituation, or repeated and purposeful moral action, enables the psychiatrist to increase visibility of virtues and obligations, and when faced with a unique situation, to more reliably practice best behavior and judgment.[5,6] Aristotle's[3] virtue-driven approach to ethics from millennia ago gained renewed interest by the twentieth century moral philosophers in the setting of virtues' accessibility and authenticity for application for plural, postmodern societies.[7,8] In other words, virtues have the potential to offer psychiatrists a more complete ethical grounding upon which to approach complex dilemmas, relative to an ad hoc, case-by-case, detached balancing act of competing interests. Virtue considerations in this article are targeted toward virtues that may be valuable in particular emergency psychiatry contexts; however, Radden and Sadler's[6] book, The Virtuous Psychiatrist, provides a much more comprehensive consideration of how virtues, or virtue ethics, can be integrated to optimize psychiatric care.

Virtue ethics is useful in the emergency psychiatry setting to aid in navigation of immense emotions and reactions such as countertransference, inconvenience while managing uncooperative patients, and constraints of time and resources. Emergency psychiatrists are frequently exposed to belligerent patient behavior, including accusations, threats, and cruel criticisms in the setting of patient agitation due to psychosis, mania, intoxication, and other presenting conditions. Virtues may guide role morality, partiality toward patients, and understanding of patient behavioral dysregulation and vulnerabilities.[4] Despite consistent caustic exposures, emergency psychiatrists must build resilience against acting on their reactions to charged patient encounters in ways that would be detrimental to their patients. Cultivating virtues is one way to counteract vices and vulnerabilities[4] and can enable professionalism in the face of even the most caustic patient behavior. For example, despite a malingering patient's discourteous behavior, externalizing accusations, and verifiable deception, the emergency psychiatrist's duty, despite the likelihood of negative reactions toward the patient and their behavior, is to perform psychiatric evaluation and management in a compassionate and respectful manner. **Table 1** lists an array of virtues relevant to the topical areas covered in this article. Habituation—practice and cultivation—of these virtues may elevate and advance ethical practice in emergency psychiatric care.

COMMON DILEMMAS IN EMERGENCY PSYCHIATRY
Competing Responsibilities to Patients and Society

Psychiatric emergencies often feature increased risk of general aggression and violence, suicide, homicide, and abuse or neglect of dependents. Patients may become vulnerable due to incapacitation from episodes of psychiatric decompensation. In these situations, the emergency psychiatrist is faced with potentially competing responsibilities for the well-being of the individual patient, as well as the greater good and safety of others in society. Emergency psychiatry, unlike many other areas of medicine, is legally circumscribed with the role of the state in addressing responsibilities to patients who need protection (parens patriae) and in preventing harm against other persons or the state itself (police power). Parens patriae represents the

Table 1
Key virtues to guide ethical practice in emergency psychiatry contexts

Context	Key Virtues
Hostile patient communication, agitation management, involuntary hospitalization	Reliability, veracity,[a] compassion, patience, tolerance and flexibility, penitence,[b] comity and courtesy,[c] reverence and deference,[d] civility, prudence and foresight, forgiveness, impartiality, courage and equanimity, restraint and tact
Collecting collateral information	Fidelity,[a] loyalty, discretion
Dilemmas in "medical clearance" evaluation	Patience, perseverance and sedulousness,[e] penitence, reverence and deference, civility, prudence, resourcefulness, and flexibility
Mandatory reporting of abuse and neglect	Sedulousness, courage, penitence, civility, detachment, discretion
Duty to warn and protect	Partiality, reliability, courage, penitence, discretion

[a] Veracity is the accuracy quality of truthfulness, whereas fidelity is the promise-keeping quality of truthfulness.
[b] Penitence is regret of wrongs and harms and desire to amend them.
[c] Comity is a harmonious and considerate effort in interactions, whereas courtesy is a considerate effort in predicting the needs of others and demonstrating polite generosity regarding these.
[d] Reverence is a formal quality of respect, whereas deference is a submissive quality of respect.
[e] Sedulousness is a motivational characteristic demonstrating attention, persistence, and careful approach to tasks of importance, whereas perseverance is persistence in a task despite presence of barriers to success.

protective role of the state and its actors, a duty to act as "parent" to care for vulnerable persons, here applied to patients incapacitated due to mental illness.[9] Parens patriae aligns with ethical principles of beneficence (to help, provide care, do good) and nonmaleficence (to not harm) as applied to psychiatric patients. Police power, on the other hand, obligates the emergency psychiatrist to manage and mitigate the potential negative impact of danger toward others that may be occasioned by the presence of mental illness.[9] Police power commands responsibility to protect a variety of stakeholders from this danger: the patient, clinical staff, general public, families and dependents of patients, and those who patients intend to physically harm. Many dilemmas arise when parens patriae and police power duties conflict with each other and with professional ethics of psychiatrists, who strive to put patient interests first and to prioritize the preferences and experiences of patients.

Confidentiality and Privacy

In the course of time-sensitive acute treatment in psychiatric emergency rooms, obtaining collateral information to inform care and maintain patient safety is often critical. Collateral information can elucidate the context of a psychiatric emergency as well as provide information relevant to assessing the risk of imminent danger. In the course of treatment, the ethical (and legal) norms for seeking and releasing information center on obtaining written informed consent before contacting sources. This standard, however, is not always feasible in psychiatric emergencies, as a patient may be too intoxicated, disorganized, agitated, or sedated to participate in the informed consent process or the patient may refuse to give permission. A patient may sometimes seek to prevent a psychiatrist's pursuit of information if attempting to avoid involuntary psychiatric admission and/or treatment, particularly if the patient has exhibited suicidal, threatening, abusive, or violent behavior and/or threats of harming themselves or others. In these situations, responsibility for patient safety and well-being may frequently conflict with respect for patient privacy. When collateral information is required to clarify a patient's imminent risk of harm to self or others, the ethical principle of beneficence weighs in favor of seeking this information. In addition, federal law (HIPAA) expressly permits collateral information to be obtained without patient consent.[10] Breaching confidentiality in these situations is not merely permissible; it is most often the standard of care that a psychiatrist will be held accountable to.[11] For example, in the 1983 case, *Jablonski v. United States*, an emergency psychiatrist warned a patient's partner to stay away from the patient, who was evaluated and diagnosed with "antisocial personality disorder." The patient made no specific threats at the time, but less than a week after discharge, he murdered his partner. The psychiatrist was found negligent in risk assessment and third-party protection due to not obtaining outside records that detailed the patient's history of schizophrenia and past attempts to kill his ex-wife.[12]

A minimal disclosure by the emergency psychiatrist is also generally permissible from a legal standpoint when collecting emergency collateral information, because it enables the contacted third party to participate in the conversation.[10] Examples of reasonable-to-disclose content include the psychiatrist's identity and credentials, a vague description of the practice setting (emergency department), and vague reassurance of the patient's well-being and safety.[11,13] *Fidelity* (promise-keeping) and *loyalty* can guide virtuous action when making judgments in these conversations. Validating the informant's emotions, educating that confidentiality standards prohibit sharing detailed updates, and advocating that the informant obtains clinical updates from the patient instead of the care team may also advance patient and informant interests.[11,13] Clearly, patient privacy is compromised in these situations to optimize nonmaleficence and beneficence to patients and society. At times, collateral information may influence the conclusion that the patient does not meet criteria for involuntary admission and can prevent the liberty constraints of psychiatric hospitalization; at other times, it may confirm the need to restrict liberties and patient-autonomous choice via involuntary psychiatric admission. As psychiatric unit beds are a scarce resource in many locales, collateral information can also promote justice through sound resource utilization when hospitalization is not clinically indicated.

Emergency psychiatrists may also seek to review patient information that is publicly available on the Internet. Such information does not fall under HIPAA protections, but concerns arise regarding privacy and vulnerability to bias by inaccurate public data.[13,14] Data sources may include court dockets, news sources, social media, mapping software, employment-related content, videos, and photographs. Suicide notes can be text messages, e-mails, or social media posts.[13] A series of questions have been proposed to clarify the ethics of patient-targeted Internet searches, the first of which is whether the search is being done to obtain clinically useful information in the patient's best interest. Patient-targeted Internet searching motivated by curiosity and voyeurism is inconsistent with professional conduct and ethics, and careful attention to the information searched and explicit identification of the need-to-know reasons for the search are ways of parsing out motivation. One investigator, for example, has compared visualizing a patient's home address in mapping software to stalking.[14] Source reliability is another consideration when seeking public domain information about patients.[13,14] Examples of relevant information that could be identified through publicly available sources include contact information for collateral sources, suicide notes, personal blogs detailing factitious or malingering content, court data regarding violent offenses, and clarification of the timing of release from legal custody.[13,14] The specific ethical considerations in the rapidly evolving digital age are a growing subject of attention and empirical study to understand expectations. For example, in a sample of forensic examinees, reviewing government Web sites was evaluated as more acceptable than reviewing social media Web sites.[15] Several investigators also advocate consideration of informed consent for Internet searches and sharing results with the patient to demonstrate integrity and honesty and to promote trust.[13,14] Documenting a justification for the search provides greater transparency and offers the opportunity for reflection on, and consideration of, the ethical standards for searches.

Nonconsensual Interventions in Acute Agitation Management

Hostility and agitation are common in psychiatric emergencies, and the psychiatrist's responsibilities to prevent harm may require coercive interventions to ensure the safety of the patient and hospital personnel alike. However, obligations to prevent harm are in tension with promotion of the patient's interest and well-being (beneficence) as well as the patient's autonomy. Humane and clinically focused agitation management balances obligations not to harm (nonmaleficence) with respect for autonomy by attempting the least invasive interventions in a graded fashion.[16] For example, high-quality verbal deescalation may avert patient psychotropic medication exposure, whether it be voluntary or involuntary. Clinical staff may optimally conduct humane verbal deescalation drawing on the particular virtues of *compassion*, *patience*, *self-control*, *civility* (polite action and expression), *deference* (humble submission), and *comity* (considerate and harmonious interaction). If verbal deescalation and psychotropic administration are insufficient to ensure safety, nonconsensual mechanical (physical) restraints may be required. The justification for the use of escalating levels of restraint is sounder when scaled, competent, lesser-intrusive measures are ineffective.

When acute agitation management requires nonconsensual interventions such as psychotropic administration and restraints, patient autonomy is clearly in conflict with preventing harm and promoting care. Hostile patient behavior and distress regarding performance of nonconsensual interventions can make agitation management a demoralizing experience for patients and clinical staff and often may not be experienced as a clinical or therapeutic intervention by either staff or the patient. In these situations, psychiatrists should reflect on their own reactions, cognitive and emotional, and review encounters with a quality improvement focus, aiming to advance clinical interventions and communication to enable promotion and optimization of future interventions. In addition, identifying the reactions of treatment staff to patients and clinical situations can assist in psychological and psychodynamic formulation of patterns of interaction. For example, countertransference of clinical team members may conjure parental (rather than clinical) mindsets toward patients, and transference of patients may project object relations from experiences with disciplinary authorities (law enforcement, parental corporal punishment) on to the clinical team. Understanding these patterns for specific patients and patients in general can inform future successful interventions.

Motivations behind agitation management interventions can also be relevant to the meaning of the clinical experience to the patient and care team. In Michael Foucault's[17] critique of early asylums (the late 1700s to the early 1800s), he observed a behavioral management approach that he called "disciplinary power." He interpreted that interventions were premised on the belief that submission and obedience can generate "the cure" of undesired behavior. These interventions were interpreted by Foucault to train patients that only constant docility and submission can earn liberty. Modern agitation management should not channel "disciplinary power," and the motivation for agitation management interventions should not be punishment or teaching lessons. Rather, the properly aligned motivation for agitation management is acute protection and harm prevention. A psychiatrist can dispel confusion about motives by maintaining awareness of power dynamics and diffusing transference or countertransference with the clear message that the interventions are "for protection and prevention, and not for punishment." To this end, the emergency psychiatrist has further responsibilities to educate and even correct team members who express the perspective that an agitated patient deserves punishment, and can provide leadership and clinical vision to model appropriate care. Actions that can deescalate problematic power dynamics in agitation management are listed in **Box 1**.

Finally, debriefing the patient is recommended after restraint placement,[16] with explanation of the indication for restraint placement and criteria for restraint deescalation. Even if the agitated patient continues hostile remarks, some degree of rapport and trust building may be enabled by a sincere and empowering debriefing. Debriefing also respects the patient by providing information and reasoning for prior invasive restraint decisions at a subsequent time at which the patient may have the requisite mental capacity to understand and/or appreciate the intervention through a different lens. In the course of a debrief, psychiatrists can also work with patients to identify patient preferences about care and future agitation management should an emergency situation again arise. Two virtues are high yield for humane debriefing. First, expression of *penitence* (acknowledging and regretting wrongs and harms toward a person, with a desire to amend them) provides an evaluation that the psychiatrist values the individual patient and commits to loyalty despite the strained patient-physician relationship. The psychiatrist can express regret that the restraints were required for

> **Box 1**
> **Action that can deescalate problematic power dynamics in agitation management**
>
> Power balancing approaches
> - Clearly communicate that interventions are "for protection and prevention, and not punishment."
> - Minimize confrontation with face-saving communication.[16,18,19]
> - Maintain open posture (do not cross arms or clench fists).[16,18]
> - Coach how to stay in control and educate on behavioral expectations.[16,19]
> - Verbalize respect and empathy.[16,18-20]
> - Position self at a 45° angle (directly in front of the patient can seem confrontational).[16,18]
> - Avoid sounding punitive or accusatory, as well as posturing to challenge.[18]
> - Give choices and encourage patient responsibility.[16,19]
> - Avoid confronting; rather, explore misconceptions.[18]
> - Deescalate security's show of force (if possible).[18]

safety, and clearly evaluate the patient for injury. Second, demonstration of *fidelity* (consistent promise keeping) can foster trust and demonstrate respect for the patient's vulnerable position. Such promises may include following through with the restraint deescalation plan and performing any indicated management for injuries or discomfort. The interaction of the aforementioned components of ethical practice in acute agitation management is depicted in **Fig. 1**.

Dilemmas in Medical Stability Evaluations

Medical clearance protocols intend to clarify what acute medical comorbidities and causes of neuropsychiatric symptoms will require management on admission to a medical or psychiatric unit. In some situations, signs, symptoms, and other contextual features may elevate the relevance of testing (ie, screening for causes of delirium in the setting of a geriatric patient with behavior change). *Persistence* and *sedulousness* (diligence and careful attention regarding important matters) are virtues that may best

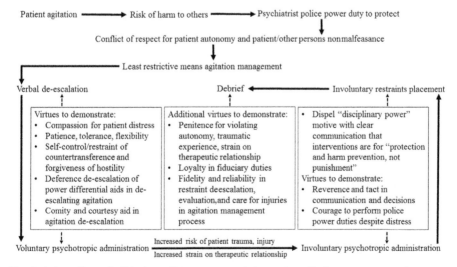

Fig. 1. Interaction of ethical practice components in acute agitation management.

enable a psychiatrist to advocate for proper care in medical clearance before a potential psychiatric admission.

Ethical dilemmas can present when a patient is uncooperative with medical clearance workup (urine and serum testing, electrocardiogram). Studies demonstrate that general medical clearance screening of patients is low yield when there is no evidence of impaired cognition before psychiatric admission,[21–23] so only targeted testing is recommended in consensus statements, with a minimum evaluation of medical stability featuring vital signs, history, physical examination, and assessment of cognition.[24,25] However, more comprehensive medical clearance testing is often a requirement for acceptance to psychiatric facilities. In a 2002 study, about one-third of the emergency department physicians surveyed reported institution-mandated medical testing for patients presenting with psychiatric emergencies.[26] In these situations, prominent considerations of justice emerge as patients may experience distress and delay in care. Waste may occur while waiting for laboratory test results, both in terms of cost and emergency room bed and resource utilization.[27] On the other hand, ensuring competent and thorough evaluation with laboratory testing as needed for patient safety cannot be abandoned.

When a patient clearly requires psychiatric admission but is not accepted by a psychiatric unit due to patient refusal of medical clearance testing, the emergency psychiatrist is put in a conflicted position. Some clinicians propose that nonconsensual medical clearance testing is supportable as an emergency intervention, under the premise that testing is necessary to facilitate the emergency intervention of psychiatric hospitalization.[28] However, this approach is not condoned in consensus recommendations[24] and could result in claims of assault and battery.[29] Optimal approaches while navigating this dilemma include demonstrating patience while negotiating with and educating the patient, building rapport in compassionate and respectful conversation, involving patient-trusted stakeholders, and conducting direct communication with the accepting psychiatrist.[1] To enable ethical practice, psychiatric units ought to have flexibility in acceptance of patients who are not suspected to have any medical instability and have been evaluated to be medically stable by an emergency medicine physician, but are uncooperative with nonessential medical clearance testing. Stratifying clearance criteria into high risk and low risk is an approach that could further deescalate potential dilemmas.[24]

Involuntary Hold and Involuntary Psychiatric Hospitalization

Psychiatric hospitalization is performed under a voluntary, conditional voluntary, or involuntary process. Conditional voluntary admission is not simply voluntary, given there are liberty-infringing strings attached. For example, patients are unable to come and go as they please and can be placed on an involuntary hold when requesting discharge to assess their safety for discharge. Conditional voluntary admission conflicts less with respect for patient autonomy, however, because informed consent must be obtained. A patient requires decision-making capacity to perform the informed consent for a conditional voluntary admission, which obligates the absence of coercion, although the law only requires a low threshold for capacitation on the sliding-scale model.[13,30] In 1990, the US Supreme Court ruled that voluntary psychiatric admission of an incapacitated patient is a deprivation of the patient's liberty "without due process of the law."[31] In other words, for situations in which a patient cannot give informed consent, treatment does not respect the person and their autonomy unless there is a capable decision maker to authorize that hospitalization or treatment. An exception is when a presently incapacitated patient has a psychiatric advanced directive (completed when capacitated) that preemptively consents to voluntary psychiatric admission in circumstances of psychiatric decompensation and incapacitation.[32,33] Specifically, in this latter scenario, the patient's autonomy is respected by virtue of honoring the prior expressed competent decision.

To be considered for involuntary psychiatric admission, there must be clear justifications for this impingement on a patient's autonomy and liberty. In general, involuntary hospitalization occurs when the patient's risk to self or others, due to mental illness, renders the hospitalization necessary to prevent harm. This approach is the dangerousness standard, which also requires that "less restrictive means" would be insufficient to manage the risk of harm.[9] Although a psychiatrist can initiate an up-to-several-day involuntary hold, lengthier involuntary psychiatric admission requires a legal (most often judicial) determination.[9] The dangerousness standard embeds a duty for societal protection primarily under the principle of state police power; however, for situations in which a patient is unable to care for themselves due to mental illness or poses a harm to themselves, the protective responsibilities of the state under *parens patriae* rationales is also implicated.[9] Finally, psychiatric advanced directives cannot avert involuntary holds for indicated involuntary admission, because they cannot negate state police power duties, despite their potential deescalation of parens patriae duties.[32]

The involuntary psychiatric admission of patients who retain decision-making capacity has been subject to critique,[34–36] including for patients intending "rational suicide."[36] Although this is an area of robust theoretic discussion, rational suicide is not currently a legally sanctioned patient right in the United States, and arrangements for medical aid in dying, in states where it is legal, are not made in the psychiatric emergency department and instead require that specific precursor steps be taken, generally including multiple steps and waiting periods.[37] In addition, some investigators propose that the efficacy of involuntary psychiatric hospitalization is insufficient to justify its burdens of nonconsensual restraint and possible medication exposures.[34,36] Yet, studies have evidenced that most patients who underwent involuntary psychiatric admissions agreed that involuntary admission was appropriate; they perceived themselves to be unwell and dangerous at the time of admission, and perceived admission to be beneficial.[38] In addition, patients who undergo involuntary hospitalization are shown to demonstrate lower social functioning before hospitalization,[39] and involuntary admission thus enables access to care for a more vulnerable population.[40] Involuntary admission can therefore promote beneficence and nonmaleficence by potentially preventing health impairment, losses (relationships, job, finances, property), and criminal justice system involvement and consequences.[40]

In addition to compromising patient autonomy, other harms experienced during involuntary psychiatric hospitalization can include stigma, shame, reenforcement of external locus of control and passivity, traumatization, damage to therapeutic alliances, and possible medication side effects.[34–36] Negative experiences voiced in surveys and interviews by patients who underwent involuntary psychiatric admission include distress regarding liberty restrictions (inability to leave, communication limitations, confiscation of property), perceived disempowerment and exclusion from decision making, disrespectful communication by personnel, coercion, and even "abusive behavior."[38,40] This clash of significant benefits and harms illustrates the challenges inherent in involuntary psychiatric care, which ought to evoke clinician *empathy*, *penitence*, and *sedulousness* when making judgments regarding involuntary psychiatric admission, and when discussing it with patients in the emergency department. Aspects prioritized by patients during involuntary admission include empowerment in decision making, general respect, respect for cultural norms and sexual orientation, and safety.[40] Furthermore, empowerment during involuntary hospitalization has been evidenced to be enhanced via provision of comprehensive education materials[41] and quality interaction with a patient's "key worker" during hospitalization.[42] Perhaps a "key worker" exhibiting virtues such as *sincerity, compassion, affability*, and *comity* contributes to these positive experiences. If so, then similar experiences in the emergency department setting may enhance care, as well.

Mandatory reporting of abuse and neglect

Screening for abuse and neglect can be easily overlooked in a fast-paced emergency care setting. Patients with cognitive impairment and intellectual disability often depend on others for resources, which makes them vulnerable to neglect and exploitation. Those with substance use may be victims of exploitation to obtain substances, and also may conduct abusive behavior when intoxicated or in withdrawal. Caregivers and parents with serious mental illness may become incapacitated, which can lead to abuse or neglect of children and vulnerable adults. Screening for the safety of patients as well as their dependents is an important facet of ethical psychiatric care and may obligate confirmation of childcare arrangements and collateral acquisition to clarify dependent safety.[13]

Although specific criteria for reporting of abuse and neglect vary by state, reporting of suspected child abuse and/or neglect is mandatory in all US jurisdictions and reporting requirements generally also cover persons with intellectual and other disability, as well as elderly persons. Information shared when reporting should be held to the standard of minimum information necessary to report the concern to respect confidentiality and patient autonomy. Disclosure of reporting obligations and reports made to authorities to patients is generally sound clinical and ethical practice in its respect for the patient,[13] and these actions require psychiatrist *courage* and humane care performed with *civility* and *penitence*. In some cases, acute risk of violence or fear of imminent danger to dependents of patients may dissuade some psychiatrists from immediately disclosing a report to a patient.[13]

Duty to protect third parties

As described previously, emergency psychiatrists inherit the societal and legal expectations that psychiatrists will act to prevent harm by patients who pose danger to others due to mental illness; this expectation includes the necessity of breaching patient confidentiality if needed to warn and protect third parties.[43] These responsibilities have emerged following the landmark California case *Tarasoff v. Regents of Univ. of California,* which established California case law placing accountability on psychiatrists to prevent harm to third parties when a patient shares intention to harm them. The 1974 decision regarding this case codified a *duty to warn* third parties; however, the California Supreme Court's 1976 decision escalated this obligation to *duty to protect* the third party.[44] This California case law has been highly influential for statues and common law in most other states.[43,45] Of note, some states have expanded psychiatrists' *duty to protect* to unspecified third parties (general public), even several months after psychiatric evaluation.[46-48] In the Vermont case *Peck v. Counseling Service of Addison County,* for example, the court ruled that psychiatrists are accountable to protect third-party property as well (a barn was burned down by a patient).[45] Psychiatrists have asserted that these extended duties and accountability are unreasonable expectations, which ignore the limitations of violence and behavior prediction.[49]

Consultation with a psychiatrist colleague or legal counsel, and documentation of consultation, can demonstrate that standard-of-care interventions are performed and also that appropriate measures were taken both to protect patient confidentiality and the public.[45] Interventions to protect third parties include patient hospitalization, warnings to police and the identified target, more frequent outpatient treatment sessions, starting or increasing the patient's medication, and various forms of closer monitoring.[45] Solely warning the identified potential victim and the police (in the precinct nearest to the patient) may be insufficient protection in some cases.[45] Some investigators propose informing the patient ahead of warning third parties, and suggest giving the patient the choice to inform the third party and police, herself.[45] Although less of a confidentiality breach by the psychiatrist, the patient may feel under coercion to perform this communication, which in turn may damage the treatment alliance. Relevant virtues here include *reliability* in the screening for dangers to third parties and *courage* to perform warnings and other protective measures, despite patient threats of litigation or revenge. *Penitent* expression of regret for the impact of warnings on a patient's distress and relationships is reasonable, and *discretion* is indicated during communication of warnings.

SUMMARY

Emergency psychiatry is rich in ethical complexity, with dilemmas often arising due to conflicts with emergency psychiatrists' competing duties to the patient and to third parties and even society. Ethical practice in these contexts may be promoted by identifying relevant ethical and legal considerations and guidance, and further optimized by the embracing virtues that supplement legal obligations and ethical principles. The dilemmas and responsibilities described herein illustrate the contemplative expertise and practical skills required for ethical practice in emergency psychiatry.

CLINICS CARE POINTS

- During agitation management, the therapeutic alliance may be buffered by modeling of therapeutic communication, communicating loyalty in duties to the patient, and sincere debriefing.
- Confidentiality should the breached in the setting of psychiatric emergencies if needed to obtain essential clinically relevant collateral information.
- Psychiatrists may be held accountable for negligence if indicated collateral information is not obtained to inform suicide or violence risk assessment.
- The legal threshold for and psychiatric hold's dangerousness standard is "clear and convincing evidence."
- Patient decision-making capacity is required for informed consent to a conditional voluntary psychiatric admission.
- Solely warning potential victims will often be inadequate in fulfilling the duty to protect persons form significant risk of harm due to a patient's mental illness.

DISCLOSURE

No personal conflicts of interest. No external funding sources.

REFERENCES

1. Allen NG, Khan JS, Alzhari MS, et al. Ethical issues in emergency psychiatry. Emerg Med Clin North Am 2015;33:863–74.

2. Beauchamp TL, Childress JF. Method and moral justification. In: Principles of biomedical ethics. 8th edition. New York: Oxford University Press; 2019. p. 425–66.
3. Tredennick H. Intellectual Virtues. In: Tredennick H. Trans, Thomson JAK, editors. The nichomachian ethics. New York: Penguin Classics; 2004. p. 144–66.
4. Radden R, Sadler JZ. Character virtues in psychiatric practice. In: Sisti DA, Caplan AL, Riman-Greenspan H, editors. Applied ethics in mental health care - an interdisciplinary reader. Cambridge (MA): MIT Press; 2013. p. 59–73.
5. Beauchamp TL, Childress JF. Moral character. In: Principles of biomedical ethics. 8th edition. New York: Oxford University Press; 2019. p. 31–64.
6. Radden R, Sadler JZ. The virtuous psychiatrist - character ethics in psychiatric practice. New York: Oxford; 2010.
7. MacIntyre A. After virtue: a study in moral theory. 3rd edition. Notre Dame (IN): University of Notre Dame Press; 2007.
8. Williams B. Ethics and the limits of philosophy. Cambridge (MA): Harvard University Press; 1986.
9. Gutheil TG, Appelbaum PS. Legal issues in emergency psychiatry. In: Clinical handbook of psychiatry and law. 4th edition. Philadelphia (PA): Lippincott Williams & Wilkens; 2007. p. 111–76.
10. Department of Health and Human Services. Health Information Portability and Accountability Act (HIPAA) Privacy Rule. 45 CFR 164.512. US.
11. Petrik ML, Billera M, Kaplan Y, et al. Balancing patient care and confidentiality: considerations in obtaining collateral information. J Psychiatr Pract 2015;21(3): 220–4.
12. Janlonski v. United States, 712 F. 2d 391 (9th Cir. 1983). case law.
13. Rajparia A. Ethical issues in emergency psychiatry. In: Maloy K, editor. A case-based approach to emergency psychiatry. New York: Oxford; 2016. p. 127–38.
14. Clinton BK, Silverman BC, Brendel DH. Patient-targeted Googling: the ethics of searching online for patient information. In: Sisti DA, Calplan AL, Rimon-Greenspan H, editors. Applied ethics in mental health care – an interdisciplinary reader. Cambridge (MA): MIT Press; 2013. p. 351–69.
15. Pirelli G, Hartigan S, Zapf PA. Using the internet for collateral information in mental health evaluations. Behav Sci Law 2018;36(2):157–69.
16. Richmond JS, Berlin JS, Fishkind AB, et al. Verbal de-escalation of the agitated patient: consensus statement of the American Association for Emergency Psychiatry Project BETA De-escalation Workshop. West J Emerg Med 2012;13(1): 17–25.
17. Foucault M. In: Larange J, Ewald F, Fontanna A, et al, editors. Psychiatric power: lectures at College de France 1973-1974. New York: Picador; 2003. p. 19–62.
18. Stevenson S. Heading off violence with verbal de-escalation. J Psychosoc Nurs Ment Health Serv 1991;29(9):6–10.
19. National Institute for Health and Care Excellence (NICE). Violence and aggression: short-term management in mental health, health and community settings NICE guideline. NG10. 2015. Available at: https://www.nice.org.uk/guidance/ng10. Accessed April 3, 2020.
20. Harwood RH. How to deal with violent and aggressive patients in medical settings. J R Coll Physicians Edinb 2017;47(2):94–101.
21. Parmar P, Goolsby CA, Udompanyanan K, et al. Value of mandatory screening studies in emergency department patients cleared for psychiatric admission. West J Emerg Med 2012;13(5):388–93.

22. Amin M, Wang J. Routine laboratory testing to evaluate for medical illness in psychiatric patients in the emergency department is largely unrevealing. West J Emerg Med 2009;10(2):97–100.
23. Gregory RJ, Nihalani ND, Rodriguez E. Medical screening in the emergency department for psychiatric admissions: a procedural analysis. Gen Hosp Psychiatry 2004;26(5):405–10.
24. Wilson MP, Nordstrom K, Anderson EL, et al. American Association for Emergency Psychiatry Task Force on Medical Clearance of Adult Psychiatric Patients. Part II: Controversies over Medical Assessment, and Consensus Recommendations. West J Emerg Med 2017;18(4):640–6.
25. Libet L, Balan Y, Thomas S. The myth of medical clearance. In: Balan Y, Murrell K, Lentz C, editors. Big book of emergency department psychiatry. Boca Raton (FL): CRC Press; 2017. p. 105–16.
26. Broderick KB, Lerner EB, McCourt JD, et al. Emergency physician practices and requirements regarding the medical screening examination of psychiatric patients. Acad Emerg Med 2002;9(1):88–92.
27. Maniaci MJ, Lachner C, Vadeboncoer TF, et al. Involuntary patient length-of-stay at a suburban emergency department. Am J Emerg Med 2020;38(3):534–8.
28. Hattem B. NYC Hospital Uses Forced Medication to Compel Bloodwork. City Limits. 2015. Available at: https://citylmits.org/2015/12/08/nyc-hospital-uses-forced -medication-to-compel-blood-work. Accessed April 14, 2020.
29. Stefan S. Legal rights and standards in emergency department treatment of people with psychiatric disabilities, . Emergency department treatment of the psychiatric patient: policy issues and legal requirements. New York: Oxford University Press; 2006.
30. Hoge SK. On being "too crazy" to sign into a mental hospital: The issue of consent to psychiatric hospitalization. Bull Am Acad Psychiatry Law 1994;22(3): 431–50.
31. Zinermon v. Burch, 494 U.S. 113 (1990). US Supreme Court case law.
32. Appelbaum P. Commentary: Psychiatric advanced directives at a crossroads – When can PADs be overwritten? J Am Acad Psychiatry Law 2006;34(3):395–7.
33. United States v. Comstock, 560 US 126, 130 S. Ct. 1949 (2010). US Supreme Court case law.
34. Hudson H. Coercion in psychiatry: is it right to involuntarily treat inpatients with capacity? J Med Ethics 2019;45(11):742–5.
35. Steinert T. Ethics of coercive treatment and misuse of psychiatry. Psychiatr Serv 2017;68:291–4.
36. Borecky A, Thomsen C, Dubov A. Reweighing the ethical tradeoffs in the involuntary hospitalization of suicidal patients. Am J Bioeth 2019;19(10):71–83.
37. Anfang S, Bonnie R, Brendel R, et al. American Psychiatric Association resource document on physician assisted death. 2017. Available at: https://www. psychiatry.org/File%20Library/Psychiatrists/Directories/Library-and-Archive/ resource_documents/2017-Resource-Document-on-Physician-Assisted-Death. pdf. Accessed August 30, 2021.
38. Valenti E, Giacco D, Katasakou C, et al. Which values are important for patients during involuntary treatment? A qualitative study with psychiatric inpatients. J Med Ethics 2014;40(12):832–6.
39. Kalbert TW, Glöckner M, Schützwhol M. Involuntary vs voluntary hospital admission: a systematic review on outcome diversity. Eur Arch Psychiatry Clin Neurosci 2017;258(4):195–209.

40. Kuosmanen L, Hätönen H, Malkavaara H, et al. Deprivation of liberty in psychiatric hospital care: The patient's perspective. Nurs Ethics 2007;14:597–607.
41. Johnsen L, Øysaed H, Barnes K, et al. A systematic intervention to improve patient information routines and satisfaction in a psychiatric emergency unit. Nord J Psychiatry 2007;61:213–8.
42. Sørgard KW. Satisfaction and coercion among voluntary, persuaded/pressured and committed patients in acute psychiatric treatment. Scand J Caring Sci 2007;21:214–9.
43. Fox PF. Commentary: so the pendulum swings – making sense of the duty to protect. J Am Acad Psychiatry Law 2010;38:474–8.
44. Tarasoff v. Regents of Univ. of Cal., 17 Cal. 3d 425, 131 Cal. Rptr. 14, 551 P.2d 334 (1976). California case law.
45. Knoll JL. The psychiatrist's duty to protect. CNS Spectr 2015;20(3):215–22.
46. Liparri v. Sears, Roebuck & Co., 497 F. Supp. 185 (D. Neb. 1980). Nebraska case law.
47. Naidu v. Laird - 539 A.2d 1064 (Del. 1988). Delaware case law.
48. Peck v. Counseling Service of Addison County, 499 A.2d 422 (1985). Vermont case law.
49. Johnson R, Persad G, Sisti D. The Tarasoff Rule: The implications of interstate variation and gaps in professional training. J Am Acad Psychiatry Law 2014; 42:469–77.

Reconsidering Gold Standards for Surrogate Decision Making for People with Dementia

James M. Wilkins, MD, DPhil[a,b,*]

KEYWORDS

- Dementia • Surrogate decision making • Capacity • Geriatric psychiatry

KEY POINTS

- With decline in cognitive functioning for persons with dementia, surrogate decision making becomes increasingly important with advancing illness.
- There are several available standards to guide surrogate decision making that can be applied in a hierarchical fashion: a person's known wishes; if there are no known previously stated wishes, then a substituted judgment can be made based on a person's previously held values and preferences; if these values and preferences are unknown, then a best-interests approach can be used.
- For people with dementia, it appears that discrepancy in proxy assessments is not only common but also associated with negative behavioral outcomes with respect to mood, relationship strain, and caregiver burden.
- In thinking about optimal approaches to proxy decision making for people with dementia, options can be offered that encourage the participation of persons with dementia either through iterative tools, such as dementia-specific advance directives and preferences assessment, or through standards that explicitly rely on consideration of longitudinal changes in values and preferences over time for persons with dementia.

INTRODUCTION

Dementia is a common neurodegenerative illness that is characterized by a progressive decline in cognitive domains, such as memory, attention, executive function, and language, that ultimately affects independent functioning with respect to activities of daily living (eg, driving, managing finances, bathing, toileting).[1] As there are several underlying pathologic conditions that can drive a dementia process, such as the

The author has nothing to disclose.
[a] Division of Geriatric Psychiatry, McLean Hospital, 115 Mill Street, Belmont, MA 02478, USA;
[b] Department of Psychiatry, Harvard Medical School, Boston, MA 02115, USA
* Division of Geriatric Psychiatry, McLean Hospital, 115 Mill Street, Belmont, MA 02478.
E-mail address: jwilkins1@partners.org

relatively common Alzheimer disease, Lewy body disease, and vascular disease, the clinical course of dementia even within a single diagnosis can be relatively heterogenous, although the advanced stages are more uniform with severe cognitive and functional impairments. Given the heterogeneity in illness progression, there tends to be a variable course of impact on decision-making capacity for people with dementia, particularly those persons at mild to moderate stages. With an inexorable decline in cognitive functioning, however, surrogate decision making becomes increasingly important and prevalent with advancing illness.[2]

For those deemed to lack decisional capacity for a decision at hand, there are several available standards to guide surrogate decision making that can be applied in a hierarchical fashion.[3] For some decisions, a person's known wishes are available through either a previous informal discussion with a surrogate or codified formally in an instructional advance directive. If there are no known previously stated wishes, then a substituted judgment can be made based on a person's previously held values and preferences; if these values and preferences are unknown, then a best-interests approach can be used.[4] A key central assumption in applying known wishes or a substituted judgment surrogate decision for a person with dementia is the presumption that these wishes, values, and preferences are stable over time and still relevant to the decision at hand.[5,6]

Unlike other incapacitating illnesses whereby there may be a clearer distinction in the transition from capacity to incapacity (eg, a catastrophic stroke), dementia is unique in that there may be a more drawn-out graying of decision-making capacity over time; indeed, median survival after a diagnosis of dementia may be up to 12 years.[1] Available data suggest that people with dementia, even those in more advanced stages, however, are generally able to reliably communicate their values and preferences and want to participate in the decision-making process, even if a surrogate is ultimately in the role of primary decision maker.[2] There is then the opportunity, in some situations, to directly compare surrogate assessments made by proxies and those made by persons with dementia themselves to see if proxies "get it right," so to speak.

The aims of this article are to highlight findings on the accuracy of surrogate assessments made in a variety of domains relevant to proxy decision making for persons with dementia, such as care, everyday psychosocial experiences, research participation, and quality of life. The importance of "getting it right" in proxy assessments with respect to autonomy for persons with dementia in applying advance directives and substituted judgments and reconsiderations of the gold-standard approach in surrogate decision making for persons with dementia are also explored.

ACCURACY OF PROXY ASSESSMENTS FOR PERSONS WITH DEMENTIA

As functional dependence increases with disease progression, aspects of personal care become a larger consideration in the day-to-day experiences of persons with dementia, even outside of more sentinel decisions, such as transitions to long-term care. Several instruments have been used to assess the values and preferences of persons with dementia. For example, the Values and Preferences Scale (VPS) was developed as a means to articulate care-related values and preferences for a person with cognitive impairment about current and future care needs.[7] In a study population of persons with mild to moderate dementia, it was found that family caregivers consistently and significantly underestimated the importance of care-related values (ie, autonomy, burden, control, family, safety) in their proxy assessments of the VPS relative to the self-reports of the study participants with dementia.[8]

Although the focus on care experiences may expand as dementia progresses, persons with dementia continue to live in a world of everyday experiences, such as daily routines, social pursuits, and leisure activities. The Preferences for Everyday Living Inventory (PELI) is a validated psychosocial preferences assessment tool for older adults comprising items across domains, such as autonomous choice, social engagement, personal growth, and keeping a routine.[9,10] In looking at the PELI as a whole in a study population of older adults with spouses as proxies, there was significantly poorer proxy agreement with self-reports of persons with dementia (Clinical Dementia Rating [CDR] score = 1) compared with those without dementia (CDR = 0).[11] Honing in further on specific PELI domains, a significant underestimation by proxy care partners was noted in the importance ratings of "social engagement" preferences (eg, regular contact with family, meeting new people, volunteering) for persons with clinically significant cognitive impairment (CDR $\geq$ 0.5).[10]

In addition, in assessing responses to treatment and other interventions for persons with cognitive impairment, in either a clinical or a research setting, proxy reports are often used to clarify the impact of an intervention and the overall health status of a person with cognitive impairment.[12] There appears, however, to be significant discrepancy in these dyadic ratings across a variety of different domains.[13] For example, in a study population of persons with Alzheimer dementia, proxy ratings by caregivers were noted to significantly underestimate quality-of-life ratings and overestimate ratings of suffering (ie, psychological, existential/spiritual, and physical) relative to the self-reports.[12] In looking at neuropsychiatric symptoms as well as quality of life in a sample of persons with mild cognitive impairment and Alzheimer dementia, proxy ratings by caregivers were noted to significantly overestimate depressive symptoms and apathy and underestimate quality of life and functional abilities relative to the self-reports.[13] Taken together, these studies suggest that social engagement, routines, and subjective experience and care values are critical to ethical and effective treatment planning for persons with dementia.

At least in part because there are currently no disease-modifying treatments available for persons with dementia and given the severity of the functional, behavioral, and financial impact of dementia, there is also tremendous pressure to elucidate better symptomatic as well as disease-modifying treatments.[14] Clinical trials are a critical means to discover novel treatments but require enrollment of persons with dementia, which can complicate the informed consent process given the actual and potential impact of cognitive impairment on decision-making capacity. As such, proxy consent has become a common practice in clinical trials involving persons with dementia to enable trial participation.[15] Within the dyad of participants with dementia and the proxy decision maker, however, there appears to be discrepancies throughout the decision-making process ranging from how the enrollment decision was made, to who ultimately made the decision to enroll, to the reasons for enrolling in the trial.[4]

IMPACTS OF DISCREPANCY IN PROXY ASSESSMENTS

The emerging evidence about person/patient-proxy decision-maker discrepancy in dementia raises questions about how to understand the impact of discrepancy in surrogate decision making and its clinical and ethical implications for people with dementia. In other words, does this discrepancy *matter*, and should we *care* about it? From a theoretic perspective, we *should* care about discrepancy in surrogate decision making. The driving bioethical principle underlying use of known wishes or a substituted judgment in proxy decision making for a person with dementia is that a person's autonomy is then preserved into the future, even in situations in which a person may be deemed incapable of making the decision at hand.[16] On this account, fundamental respect for persons and humanity would require that more be done to align decisions made on behalf of incapacitated persons with their actual preferences, values, and wishes. In addition, a stronger sense of autonomy appears to be an important predictor of life satisfaction for older adults as well as a predictor of lower levels of depression and agitation,[17] thereby adding additional clinical evidence in support of this ethical stance. Thus, at least from a general, theoretic, and statistical standpoint, processes that reduce the sense of autonomy do have negative impacts on perceived quality of life as well as neuropsychiatric experiences for persons with cognitive impairment.

That being said, it is not always clear to what extent, if any, a statistical relationship will correlate with an appreciable clinical difference. It does appear, however, that discrepancies in proxy assessments are associated with significant clinical differences in some situations. For instance, a higher level of discrepancy between proxy ratings and self-reports on the importance of "social engagement" preferences was significantly associated with increasing depressive symptoms for persons with clinically significant cognitive impairment.[10] With respect to socioemotional care preferences (ie, companionship, activities, going out, emotional support), discrepancy between proxy assessments and self-reports for persons with dementia was also significantly associated with reports of greater dyadic relationship strain as well as worse mood for the person with dementia.[18] In addition, caregiver burden was associated with discrepancy between proxy assessments and self-reports of quality of life for persons with Alzheimer dementia,[12] highlighting the importance of focusing on all members of the patient-caregiver dyads and caregiver teams to align care and treatment.

APPROACHES TOWARD OPTIMIZING SURROGATE DECISION MAKING FOR PERSONS WITH DEMENTIA

Although a substituted judgment is considered the gold-standard approach to surrogate decision making and, in some instances the legally recommended (and even required) approach, proxy decision makers do not necessarily follow these guidelines in decisions for persons with dementia.[19] For instance, in a study of proxy decisions made by family members for persons with advanced Alzheimer dementia, proxies appeared to preferentially use a best-interests approach instead of a substituted judgment approach in medical decision making.[20] Thus, in addition to the discrepancies in accurately applying a substituted judgment as described above when it is applied, there appears to be a disconnect in the theoretic recommendations, ethical guidance, and legal standard and the practical approaches taken by proxies for persons with dementia.

In order to faithfully implement and optimize surrogate decision making for persons with dementia, then, one could consider several avenues to address the discrepancies in assessment of values and preferences as well as the method of making proxy decisions. First, in keeping with the core assumption of preferential status for a substituted judgment approach because it most closely approximates the person's own autonomous decision were the person competent, efforts could be made to improve the fidelity in proxy assessments. From a purely theoretic standpoint, a substituted judgment would be made as follows: a decision is to be made; a person with dementia is deemed to lack capacity to make that decision; a surrogate decision maker is sought; the surrogate uses an understanding of the person's past preferences and values to make the decision, thus preserving the autonomy of the person with dementia into the future. This approach could be strengthened by recognizing that a proxy decision for a person with dementia does not necessarily have to be focused on the past or a grab-back into a vacuum of some prior conversation or experience. Instead, given the heterogeneity of dementia processes and their clinical courses, there may be ample opportunities for a proxy to review values and preferences with a person with dementia over time and into the future, particularly given that values and preferences may fundamentally change over time in the face of a life-altering diagnosis and illness.[6]

Akin to the process of advance care planning more generally, a review of the values and preferences of a person with dementia can (and should) be an iterative process over time, allowing flexibility and evolution in the setting of changing life circumstances[21] and the ability to assess and modify treatment plans and goals for care over time. With respect to health care decisions, a dementia-specific advance directive has been suggested to focus on goal-directed discussions in the context of various clinical stages of a progressive illness.[22] This recommendation could inform and support an iterative, flexible, and person-centered approach to decision making within person-proxy dyads and systems to promote both the autonomy and the quality of life for people with dementia. Beyond health care decisions, the importance of individual values has also led to a greater focus on incorporating psychosocial preferences into the everyday experiences of people with dementia, particularly those in long-term care settings, using assessments similar to the PELI to maximize person-centered approaches.[23] The consequence here is the recognition that substituted judgments and proxy decision making are best conceptualized and can be optimized through a forward-looking, dynamic, and inclusive approach of refining preferences assessments using structured tools that rely on direct contributions from persons with cognitive impairment and a present-informed view toward the future rather than through overreliance on historical data and perspectives.

A further consideration in optimizing surrogate decision making for persons with dementia would be a deemphasis of the standard hierarchy of proxy approaches altogether. For instance, some proxy decision makers see no substantive difference between a substituted judgment and best-interests approach in medical decision making for people with dementia.[20] In looking at proxy medical decision making more generally outside of cognitive impairment per se, it appears that this standard hierarchy of proxy approaches is often ignored by proxies, clinicians, and even patients themselves.[3] The question remains then whether these standard approaches for proxy decision making are meaningful and useful at all in the unique context of dementia. Instead of parsing through standards with apparent limited utility and effectiveness, attention could be more constructively and ethically focused on concepts and methods that have actual clinical and quality-of-life import and maximize respect for the changing perspectives and experiences of people with dementia during the course of their illness through even limited participation in decision making.

Previously, the authors have argued that a dementia-specific standard for surrogate decision making is needed given the inflexibility of substituted judgments and the subjectivity in best-interests assessments for people with dementia.[6] A narrative interest standard has been advanced for surrogate decision making for people with dementia in which there is a focus on the risks/benefits of a decision at hand while incorporating a narrative review with space for the direct contributions of a person with dementia to provide further context and flexibility for values and preferences over time.[6] The foundational piece of this approach is the opportunity for the person with dementia to participate in the decision-making process, particularly in those settings where a proxy is the designated primary decision maker.

SUMMARY

As the cognitive impairments inherent to dementia progress, surrogate decision making becomes an increasingly active part in the life of a person with dementia. By convention, there is a hierarchical approach to proxy decision making with known wishes, then a substituted judgment standard, and then a best-interests standard. For people with dementia, it appears that discrepancy in proxy assessments is not only common but also associated with negative behavioral outcomes with respect to mood, relationship strain, and caregiver burden. In thinking about optimal approaches to proxy decision making for people with dementia, options can be offered that encourage the participation of persons with dementia either through iterative tools, such as dementia-specific advance directives and preferences assessment, or through standards that explicitly rely on consideration of longitudinal changes in values and preferences over time for persons with dementia.

CLINICS CARE POINTS

- It appears that people with dementia, even those in more advanced stages, are generally able to reliably communicate their values and preferences and want to participate in the decision-making process, even if a surrogate is ultimately in the role of primary decision maker.

- It appears that discrepancy in proxy assessments for persons with dementia is not only common but also associated with negative behavioral outcomes with respect to mood, relationship strain, and caregiver burden.

- In thinking about optimal approaches to proxy decision making for people with dementia, options can be recommended that encourage the participation of persons with dementia either through iterative tools, such as dementia-specific advance directives and preferences assessment, or through standards that explicitly rely on consideration of longitudinal changes in values and preferences over time for persons with dementia.

ACKNOWLEDGEMENTS

This work was supported by an Alzheimer's Association Clinician Scientist Fellowship (JMW) and National Institutes of Health Loan Repayment Award, L30 AG060475 (JMW).

REFERENCES

1. Mitchell SL. Advanced dementia. N Engl J Med 2015;372(26):2533–40.
2. Miller LM, Whitlatch CJ, Lyons KS. Shared decision-making in dementia: a review of patient and family carer involvement. Dementia 2016;15(5):1141–57.
3. Berger JT, DeRenzo EG, Schwartz J. Surrogate decision making: reconciling ethical theory and clinical practice. Ann Intern Med 2008;149(1):48–53.
4. Black BS, Wechsler M, Fogarty L. Decision making for participation in dementia research. Am J Geriatr Psychiatry 2013;21(4):355–63.
5. Holm S. Autonomy, authenticity, or best interest: everyday decision-making and persons with dementia. Med Health Care Philos 2001;4(2):153–9.
6. Wilkins JM. Narrative interest standard: a novel approach to surrogate decision-making for people with dementia. Gerontologist 2018;58(6):1016–20.
7. Whitlatch CJ, Feinberg LF, Tucke SS. Measuring the values and preferences for everyday care of persons with cognitive impairment and their family caregivers. Gerontologist 2005;45(3):370–80.

8. Reamy AM, Kim K, Zarit SH, et al. Understanding discrepancy in perceptions of values: individuals with mild to moderate dementia and their family caregivers. Gerontologist 2011;51(4):473–83.
9. Van Haitsma K, Curyto K, Spector A, et al. The preferences for everyday living inventory: scale development and description of psychosocial preferences responses in community-dwelling elders. Gerontologist 2013;53(4):582–95.
10. Wilkins JM, Locascio JJ, Gunther JM, et al. Differences in assessment of everyday preferences between people with cognitive impairment and their care partners: the role of neuropsychiatric symptoms. Am J Geriatr Psychiatry 2020; 28(10):1070–8.
11. Carpenter BD, Kissel EC, Lee MM. Preferences and life evaluations of older adults with and without dementia: reliability, stability, and proxy knowledge. Psychol Aging 2007;22(3):650–5.
12. Schulz R, Cook TB, Beach SR, et al. Magnitude and causes of bias among family caregivers rating Alzheimer disease patients. Am J Geriatr Psychiatry 2013;21(1): 14–25.
13. Pfeifer L, Drobetz R, Fankhauser S, et al. Caregiver rating bias in mild cognitive impairment and mild Alzheimer's disease: impact of caregiver burden and depression on dyadic rating discrepancy across domains. Int Psychogeriatr 2013;25(8):1345–55.
14. Wilkins JM, Forester BP. Informed consent, therapeutic misconception, and clinical trials for Alzheimer's disease. Int J Geriatr Psychiatry 2020;35(5):430–5.
15. De Vries R, Ryan KA, Stanczyk A, et al. Public's approach to surrogate consent for dementia research: cautious pragmatism. Am J Geriatr Psychiatry 2013; 21(4):364–72.
16. Tenenbaum E. To be or to exist: standards for deciding whether dementia patients in nursing homes should engage in intimacy, sex, and adultery. Indiana L Rev 2009;42(15):675–721.
17. Wright JL. Guardianship for your own good: improving the well-being of respondents and wards in the USA. Int J L Psychiatry 2010;33(5–6):350–68.
18. Shelton EG, Orsulic-Jeras S, Whitlatch CJ, et al. Does it matter if we disagree? The impact of incongruent care preferences on persons with dementia and their care partners. Gerontologist 2018;58(3):556–66.
19. Dunn LB, Fisher SR, Hantke M, et al. "Thinking about it for somebody else": Alzheimer's disease research and proxy decision makers' translation of ethical principles into practice. Am J Geriatr Psychiatry 2013;21(4):337–45.
20. Hirschman KB, Kapo JM, Karlawish JHT. Why doesn't a family member of a person with advanced dementia use a substituted judgment when making a decision for that person? Am J Geriatr Psychiatry 2006;14(8):659–67.
21. Inoue M, Moorman SM. Does end-of-life planning help partners become better surrogates? Gerontologist 2015;55(6):951–60.
22. Gaster B, Larson EB, Curtis JR. Advance directives for dementia. JAMA 2017; 318(22):2175.
23. Van Haitsma K, Abbott KM, Arbogast A, et al. A preference-based model of care: an integrative theoretical model of the role of preferences in person-centered care. Gerontologist 2020;60(3):376–84.

UNITED STATES POSTAL SERVICE ® — Statement of Ownership, Management, and Circulation (All Periodicals Publications Except Requester Publications)

1. Publication Title	2. Publication Number	3. Filing Date
PSYCHIATRIC CLINICS OF NORTH AMERICA	000 – 703	9/18/2021

4. Issue Frequency	5. Number of Issues Published Annually	6. Annual Subscription Price
MAR, JUN, SEP, DEC	4	$338.00

7. Complete Mailing Address of Known Office of Publication *(Not printer) (Street, city, county, state, and ZIP+4®)*
ELSEVIER INC.
230 Park Avenue, Suite 800
New York, NY 10169

Contact Person
Malathi Samayan

Telephone *(Include area code)*
91-44-4299-4507

8. Complete Mailing Address of Headquarters or General Business Office of Publisher *(Not printer)*
ELSEVIER INC.
230 Park Avenue, Suite 800
New York, NY 10169

9. Full Names and Complete Mailing Addresses of Publisher, Editor, and Managing Editor *(Do not leave blank)*

Publisher *(Name and complete mailing address)*
DOLORES MELONI, ELSEVIER INC.
1600 JOHN F KENNEDY BLVD. SUITE 1800
PHILADELPHIA, PA 19103-2899

Editor *(Name and complete mailing address)*
LAUREN BOYLE, ELSEVIER INC.
1600 JOHN F KENNEDY BLVD. SUITE 1800
PHILADELPHIA, PA 19103-2899

Managing Editor *(Name and complete mailing address)*
PATRICK MANLEY, ELSEVIER INC.
1600 JOHN F KENNEDY BLVD. SUITE 1800
PHILADELPHIA, PA 19103-2899

10. Owner *(Do not leave blank. If the publication is owned by a corporation, give the name and address of the corporation immediately followed by the names and addresses of all stockholders owning or holding 1 percent or more of the total amount of stock. If not owned by a corporation, give the names and addresses of the individual owners. If owned by a partnership or other unincorporated firm, give its name and address as well as those of each individual owner. If the publication is published by a nonprofit organization, give its name and address.)*

Full Name	Complete Mailing Address
WHOLLY OWNED SUBSIDIARY OF REED/ELSEVIER, US HOLDINGS	1600 JOHN F KENNEDY BLVD. SUITE 1800 PHILADELPHIA, PA 19103-2899

11. Known Bondholders, Mortgagees, and Other Security Holders Owning or Holding 1 Percent or More of Total Amount of Bonds, Mortgages, or Other Securities. If none, check box ▶ ☐ None

Full Name	Complete Mailing Address
N/A	

12. Tax Status *(For completion by nonprofit organizations authorized to mail at nonprofit rates) (Check one)*
The purpose, function, and nonprofit status of this organization and the exempt status for federal income tax purposes:
☒ Has Not Changed During Preceding 12 Months
☐ Has Changed During Preceding 12 Months *(Publisher must submit explanation of change with this statement)*

PS Form 3526, July 2014 *[Page 1 of 4 (see instructions page 4)]* PSN 7530-01-000-9931   PRIVACY NOTICE: See our privacy policy on www.usps.com

---

13. Publication Title		14. Issue Date for Circulation Data Below
PSYCHIATRIC CLINICS OF NORTH AMERICA		JUNE 2021

15. Extent and Nature of Circulation			Average No. Copies Each Issue During Preceding 12 Months	No. Copies of Single Issue Published Nearest to Filing Date
a. Total Number of Copies *(Net press run)*			204	160
b. Paid Circulation *(By Mail and Outside the Mail)*	(1)	Mailed Outside-County Paid Subscriptions Stated on PS Form 3541 (Include paid distribution above nominal rate, advertiser's proof copies, and exchange copies)	98	81
	(2)	Mailed In-County Paid Subscriptions Stated on PS Form 3541 (Include paid distribution above nominal rate, advertiser's proof copies, and exchange copies)	0	0
	(3)	Paid Distribution Outside the Mails Including Sales Through Dealers and Carriers, Street Vendors, Counter Sales, and Other Paid Distribution Outside USPS®	65	50
	(4)	Paid Distribution by Other Classes of Mail Through the USPS (e.g., First-Class Mail®)	0	0
c. Total Paid Distribution *(Sum of 15b (1), (2), (3), and (4))*		▶	163	131
d. Free or Nominal Rate Distribution *(By Mail and Outside the Mail)*	(1)	Free or Nominal Rate Outside-County Copies included on PS Form 3541	25	13
	(2)	Free or Nominal Rate In-County Copies Included on PS Form 3541	0	0
	(3)	Free or Nominal Rate Copies Mailed at Other Classes Through the USPS (e.g., First-Class Mail)	0	0
	(4)	Free or Nominal Rate Distribution Outside the Mail (Carriers or other means)	0	0
e. Total Free or Nominal Rate Distribution *(Sum of 15d (1), (2), (3) and (4))*		▶	25	13
f. Total Distribution *(Sum of 15c and 15e)*		▶	188	144
g. Copies not Distributed *(See Instructions to Publishers #4 (page 3))*		▶	16	16
h. Total *(Sum of 15f and g)*		▶	204	160
i. Percent Paid *(15c divided by 15f times 100)*			86.7%	90.97%

* If you are claiming electronic copies, go to line 16 on page 3. If you are not claiming electronic copies, skip to line 17 on page 3.

16. Electronic Copy Circulation		Average No. Copies Each Issue During Preceding 12 Months	No. Copies of Single Issue Published Nearest to Filing Date
a. Paid Electronic Copies	▶		
b. Total Paid Print Copies (Line 15c) + Paid Electronic Copies (Line 16a)	▶		
c. Total Print Distribution (Line 15f) + Paid Electronic Copies (Line 16a)	▶		
d. Percent Paid (Both Print & Electronic Copies) (16b divided by 16c × 100)	▶		

☒ I certify that 50% of all my distributed copies (electronic and print) are paid above a nominal price.

17. Publication of Statement of Ownership
☒ If the publication is a general publication, publication of this statement is required. Will be printed in the ___DECEMBER 2021___ issue of this publication.   ☐ Publication not required.

18. Signature and Title of Editor, Publisher, Business Manager, or Owner

Malathi Samayan - Distribution Controller   *Malathi Samayan*   Date 9/18/2021

I certify that all information furnished on this form is true and complete. I understand that anyone who furnishes false or misleading information on this form or who omits material or information requested on the form may be subject to criminal sanctions (including fines and imprisonment) and/or civil sanctions (including civil penalties).

PS Form 3526, July 2014 *(Page 3 of 4)*   PRIVACY NOTICE: See our privacy policy on www.usps.com

Moving?

Make sure your subscription moves with you!

To notify us of your new address, find your **Clinics Account Number** (located on your mailing label above your name), and contact customer service at:

Email: journalscustomerservice-usa@elsevier.com

800-654-2452 (subscribers in the U.S. & Canada)
314-447-8871 (subscribers outside of the U.S. & Canada)

Fax number: 314-447-8029

Elsevier Health Sciences Division
Subscription Customer Service
3251 Riverport Lane
Maryland Heights, MO 63043

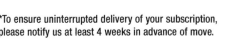

*To ensure uninterrupted delivery of your subscription, please notify us at least 4 weeks in advance of move.

ELSEVIER

Printed and bound by CPI Group (UK) Ltd, Croydon, CR0 4YY

03/10/2024

01040480-0016